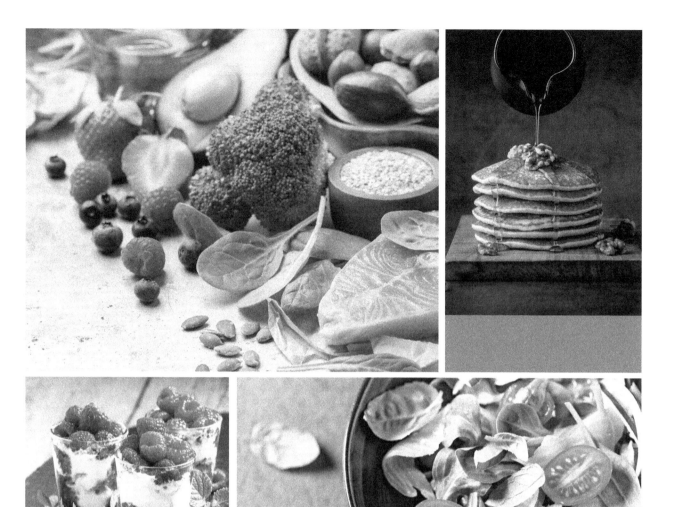

KETO DIET FOR WOMEN AFTER 50

THE ULTIMATE EASY & HEALTHY RECIPES FOR WEIGHT LOSS,
BALANCING HORMONES AND FEELING GREAT | 30-DAY MEAL PLAN INCLUDED

Suzanne Busy

Copyright - 2020 -

All rights reserved.

The content contained within this book may not be reproduced, duplicated or transmitted without direct written permission from the author or the publisher.

Under no circumstances will any blame or legal responsibility be held against the publisher, or author, for any damages, reparation, or monetary loss due to the information contained within this book. Either directly or indirectly.

Legal Notice:

This book is copyright protected. This book is only for personal use. You cannot amend, distribute, sell, use, quote or paraphrase any part, or the content within this book, without the consent of the author or publisher.

Disclaimer Notice:

Please note the information contained within this document is for educational and entertainment purposes only. All effort has been executed to present accurate, up to date, and reliable, complete information. No warranties of any kind are declared or implied. Readers acknowledge that the author is not engaging in the rendering of legal, financial, medical or professional advice. The content within this book has been derived from various sources. Please consult a licensed professional before attempting any techniques outlined in this book.

By reading this document, the reader agrees that under no circumstances is the author responsible for any losses, direct or indirect, which are incurred as a result of the use of information contained within this document, including, but not limited to, - errors, omissions, or inaccuracies.

TABLE OF CONTENTS

INTRODUCTION
6

1. WHY KETO: BENEFITS OF THE KETOGENIC DIET FOR PEOPLE OVER 50
8

2. HOW TO KNOW YOU ARE IN KETOSIS
12

3. WHAT DOES THE KETOGENIC DIET MEAN FOR WOMEN AFTER 50?
16

4. THE ULTIMATE KETO SHOPPING LIST
20

5. MENOPAUSE AND THE KETOGENIC DIET
24

6. BREAKFAST
26

- CHEESE CREPES
  27

- RICOTTA PANCAKES
  28

- YOGURT WAFFLES
  29

- BROCCOLI MUFFINS
  30

- PUMPKIN BREAD
  31

- EGGS IN AVOCADO CUPS
  32

- CHEDDAR SCRAMBLE
  33

- BACON OMELET

34

- GREEN VEGGIES QUICHE — 35
- CHICKEN & ASPARAGUS FRITTATA — 36

7. LUNCH — 38

- KETO BURGER FAT BOMBS — 39
- KETO TACO CUPS — 40
- CAPRESE ZOODLES — 41
- ZUCCHINI SUSHI — 42
- ASIAN CHICKEN LETTUCE WRAPS — 43
- PROSCIUTTO AND MOZZARELLA BOMB — 44
- KETOFIED CHICK-FIL-A-STYLE CHICKEN — 45
- CHEESEBURGER TOMATOES — 46

8. DINNER — 48

- KORMA CURRY — 49
- ZUCCHINI BARS — 50
- MUSHROOM SOUP — 51
- STUFFED PORTOBELLO MUSHROOMS — 52
- LETTUCE SALAD — 53
- ONION SOUP — 54
- ASPARAGUS SALAD — 55
- BEEF WITH CABBAGE NOODLES — 56
- ROAST BEEF AND MOZZARELLA PLATE — 57
- GARLIC HERB BEEF ROAST — 58
- SPROUTS STIR-FRY WITH KALE, BROCCOLI, AND BEEF — 59
- BEEF AND VEGETABLE SKILLET — 60
- BEEF, PEPPER AND GREEN BEANS STIR-FRY — 61

9. MEAT RECIPES — 62

- BEEF WITH CABBAGE NOODLES — 63
- ROAST BEEF AND MOZZARELLA PLATE — 64

- BEEF AND BROCCOLI — 65
- GARLIC HERB BEEF ROAST — 66
- SPROUTS STIR-FRY WITH KALE, BROCCOLI, AND BEEF — 67
- BEEF AND VEGETABLE SKILLET — 68
- BEEF, PEPPER AND GREEN BEANS STIR-FRY — 69
- CHEESY MEATLOAF — 70
- ROAST BEEF AND VEGETABLE PLATE — 71
- STEAK AND CHEESE PLATE — 72
- GARLICKY STEAKS WITH ROSEMARY — 73

10. FISH SEAFOOD — 74
- SWEET & SOUR GROUPER — 75
- AROMATIC COD — 76
- FLAVORSOME COD BAKE — 77
- SUPER-SIMPLE TROUT — 78

11. SNACKS — 80
- KORMA CURRY — 81
- COCONUT FUDGE — 82
- NUTMEG NOUGAT — 83
- SWEET ALMOND BITES — 84
- STRAWBERRY CHEESECAKE MINIS — 85
- COCOA BROWNIES — 86
- CHOCOLATE ORANGE BITES — 87
- CARAMEL CONES — 88
- CINNAMON BITES — 89
- SWEET CHAI BITES — 90
- EASY VANILLA BOMBS — 91
- MARINATED EGGS — 92
- SAUSAGE AND CHEESE DIP — 93
- TASTY ONION AND CAULIFLOWER DIP — 94

- PESTO CRACKERS — 95
- PUMPKIN MUFFINS — 96

12. DESSERT — 98
- SUGAR-FREE LEMON BARS — 99
- CREAMY HOT CHOCOLATE — 100
- DELICIOUS COFFEE ICE CREAM — 101
- FATTY BOMBS WITH CINNAMON AND CARDAMOM — 102
- EASY PEANUT BUTTER CUPS — 103
- RASPBERRY MOUSSE — 104
- CHOCOLATE SPREAD WITH HAZELNUTS — 105
- QUICK AND SIMPLE BROWNIE — 106
- CUTE PEANUT BALLS — 107
- CHOCOLATE MUG MUFFINS — 108

13. CONDIMENTS, SAUCES, & SPREADS RECIPES — 110
- CURRY POWDER — 111
- POULTRY SEASONING — 112
- BBQ SAUCE — 113
- KETCHUP — 114
- CRANBERRY SAUCE — 115
- KETCHUP — 116
- YOGURT TZATZIKI — 117

14. 30-DAY MEAL PLAN — 118

15. PROHIBITED PRODUCTS LIST — 122

CONCLUSION — 126

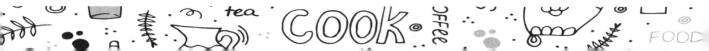

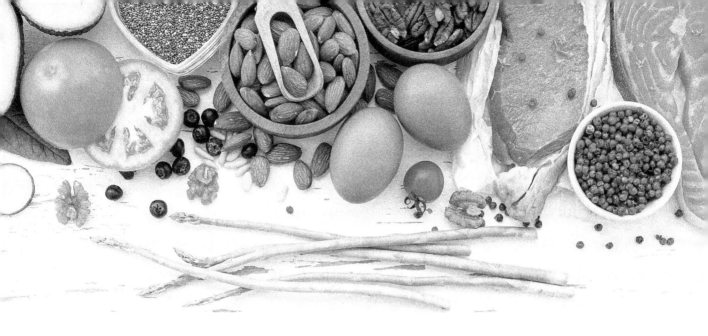

INTRODUCTION

The Keto diet has received great appreciation and praise for its weight loss benefits. This high-fat, low-carbohydrate diet has been shown to be extremely healthy overall. It really makes your body burn fat, like a machine. Public figures also appreciate it. But the question is, how does ketosis improve weight loss? Here is a detailed picture of the ketosis and weight loss process.

Ketosis is considered abnormal by some people. Although it has been approved by many nutritionists and doctors, many people still disapprove of it. The misconceptions are due to the myths that have spread around the ketogenic diet.

Once your body has no glucose, it will automatically depend on the stored fat. It is also important to understand that carbohydrates produce glucose, and once you start a low carb diet, you will also be able to lower your glucose levels. Then your body is going to create fuel through fats, instead of carbohydrates, that is, glucose.

The process of creating fat through fat is known as ketosis, and once your body enters this state, it becomes extremely effective in burning unwanted fat. Also, since glucose levels are low during the keto diet, your body achieves many other health benefits.

A ketogenic diet is not only beneficial for weight loss, it also helps improve your overall health in a positive way. Unlike all other diet plans, which focus on reducing calorie intake, keto emphasizes putting your body in a natural metabolic state, namely ketosis. The only factor that makes this diet plan questionable is that this nature of metabolism is not much deliberated. With your body making ketones regularly, your body will quickly burn stored fat, leading to great weight loss.

Now the question arises. How does ketosis

affect the human body?

The truth is, a Keto diet is healthy for almost everyone. However, we must accept that this diet plan is completely different from what we usually try. Your body will definitely react a little to the new process. The side effects are called "Keto-flu," during which one may experience extreme hunger, low energy levels, lack of sleep, and nausea.

However, this phase does not last more than 2-3 days. This is the time it takes for the human body to enter the ketosis phase. Once you enter it, you will not have any adverse side effects.

Also, you should gradually start reducing your calorie and carbohydrate intake. The most common mistake dietitians make is that they tend to start eliminating everything from their diet at the same time. This is where the problem arises. The human body will react extremely negatively when you limit everything at once. You need to start gradually. Read this guide for more information on how to approach the keto diet after 50.

Most fats are good and are essential to our health that's why there are essential fatty acids and essential amino acids (protein). Fats are the most efficient form of energy, and each gram contains about 9 calories. That's more than double the amount in carbohydrates and protein (both have 4 calories per gram).

When you eat a lot of fat and protein and drastically reduce carbohydrates, your body adapts and converts the fat and protein, as well as the fat that it has stored, into ketones or ketones for energy. This metabolic process is called ketosis. That's where the ketogenic diet comes from.

1. WHY KETO: BENEFITS OF THE KETOGENIC DIET FOR PEOPLE OVER 50

We all know that our body needs energy for its functioning, and the energy sources come from carbohydrates, proteins, and fats. Owing to years of conditioning that a low-fat carbohydrate-rich diet is essential for good health, we have become used to depending on glucose (from carbohydrates) to get most of the energy that our body needs. Only when the amount of glucose available for energy generation decreases does our body begin to break down fat for drawing energy to power our cells and organs. This is the express purpose of a ketogenic diet.

The primary aim of a ketogenic diet (also called the Keto diet) is to convert your body into a fat-burning machine. Such a diet is loaded with benefits and is highly recommended by nutritional experts for the following results:

- Natural appetite control
- Increased mental clarity
- Lowered levels of inflammation in the body system
- Improved stability in blood sugar levels
- Elimination or lower risk of heartburn
- Using natural stored body fat as the fuel source
- Weight loss

The effects listed are just some of the numerous impacts that take place when a person embarks on a ketogenic diet and makes it a point to stick to it. A ketogenic diet consists of meals with low carbohydrates, moderate proteins, and high-fat content. The mechanism works like this: when we drastically reduce the intake of carbohydrates, our body is compelled to convert fat for releasing energy. This process of converting fats instead of carbohydrates to release energy is called Ketosis.

Health Benefits of Keto Diet to Women Above 50

Both low-fat and also low-carb diet plans can be reliable for weight loss, according to the American Association of Retired Persons (AARP). The low-carb diet has some extra health and wellness advantages worth taking into consideration. The researcher also went so far as to recommend that the low-carb diet plan might provide a choice to pain-relieving opioids.

Besides, low-carb diet plans might aid HDL (good) cholesterol and triglyceride degrees much more efficiently than even more carb-heavy diet plans, according to the Mayo Clinic. Today, low-carb diet plans have taken several popular types, consisting of the Keto diet plan, the Paleo diet plan, and the Mediterranean diet. While each of these choices includes its nuances, they're all based around lowering carbohydrate intake while raising healthy and balanced fat consumption.

Decreased Thyroid Function

A research study has discovered that a ketogenic diet plan lowers the degree of T3, the body's active thyroid hormonal agent. Unfortunately, this suggests a ketogenic diet might not be optimal for those with preexisting hypothyroidism. Consult with your physician first since you may require thyroid assistance if you have hypothyroidism and want to continue with a ketogenic diet plan.

Elevated Cortisol

A research study has suggested that a ketogenic diet plan raises the tension hormonal agent cortisol to increase power levels despite reduced carbohydrate availability. It is still debated whether this increase in cortisol is harmless or dangerous. Getting a lot of rest, exercising, and engaging in a routine stress-reduction technique can assist you in keeping your standard tension degrees reduced and decrease the possibility for consistently elevated cortisol.

- Nutrient deficiencies: Older grownups often tend to have more significant shortages in essential nutrients like:
- Iron: the deficiency can lead to mental fog and also exhaustion
- Vitamin B12: deficiency can cause neurological problems like dementia.
- Fats: deficiency can lead to troubles with cognition, vitamin, vision, and even skin shortages.
- Vitamin D: deficiency can cause cognitive problems in older grownups, raise the danger of cardiovascular disease, and also contribute to cancer cells threat. The top-quality resources of animal protein on the ketogenic diet plan can quickly account for excellent sources of these essential nutrients.

Regulating Blood Sugar

As we've talked about, the connection between low blood sugar and also associated brain circumstances like Alzheimer's disease, mental weakening, and Parkinson's disease exists. Excess consumption of carbohydrates, mainly from fructose, will be drastically lowered in the ketogenic diet.

An absence of nutritional fats and cholesterol-- which are bountiful and also healthy and balanced on the ketogenic diet plan.

Making use of a ketogenic diet to assist in regulating blood sugar levels and improve nourishment might assist not only improve insulin response but also secure against memory issues that frequently come with age.

Keto foods provide a high amount of nutrition per calorie. This is crucial because basal metabolic rate (the number of calories needed daily to endure) is less for seniors. Yet, they still need the same quantity of nutrients as younger people.

A person age 50+ will have a much more challenging time residing on junk foods than a teenager or 20+ whose body is still resilient. This makes it also a lot more critical for seniors to eat foods that are disease-fighting and health-supporting. It can necessarily imply the difference between enjoying the golden years to the max or spending them suffering and in pain.

Older women should eat a much better diet plan by avoiding "empty calories" from sugars or nutrient-dense foods such as whole grains and also increasing the amount of healthy, nutrient-rich proteins. Additionally, much of the food chosen by older people (or given up medical facility or clinical settings) often tend to be significantly refined and very poor in nutrients, such as white bread, pasta, prunes, mashed potatoes, puddings, and so on.

It's quite clear that the high-carb diet so commonly pushed by the government is not best for sustaining our senior women and also their lasting health and wellness. A diet plan low in carbs and abundant in animal and plant fats are much better for promoting a much better insulin level of sensitivity, and also overall better health and wellness.

Ketosis for Longevity

That being said, the earlier we can start making changes that support healthy and balanced weight, blood sugar, immunity, and extra, the greater the chance of having less pain and suffering later on in life. Note: We're all growing older, and death is, naturally, unavoidable. People are currently living much longer; however, we're additionally getting sicker by complying with the typical diet plan of the majority. The ketogenic diet can help elders boost their wellness so that they can grow, instead of being ill or hurting during the later years of life.

Because your body turns fat from your diet plan and your inner fat shops into ketones, the keto diet rapidly enhances weight loss. And also, ketones cannot be stored as fat since they aren't digested similarly.

It's incredible; for years, you've heard that fat makes you gain weight. Your body has evolved to use fat as a different source of energy. For most of history, people did not eat three meals and snacks all day.

2. HOW TO KNOW YOU ARE IN KETOSIS

As you practice the ketogenic diet further, you will be able to tell you are in Ketosis through the signs and symptoms you are going to experience. Remember that you will now be providing your body with a new fuel source. It is going to take a little bit of time to adapt your body to this change. Below, you will find the most common symptoms of Ketosis to tell if you are following the diet correctly.

Bad Breath

I know, a great introduction to the ketogenic diet, but bad breath is one of the most reported symptoms for individuals who have reached full Ketosis. The good news is that this is a widespread side effect for individuals who follow a low-carb diet. Some have described the scent as a "fruit" smell.

Elevated ketone levels in your body cause this scent. The smell is the acetone that exits your body through breath and urine. And while this symptom is less than ideal for your friends and family, it is an excellent sign that you are following your diet correctly! To solve this issue, you will want to brush your teeth a few times a day or find a sugar-free gum to chew on.

Increased Ketones in Blood, Urine, or Breath

As mentioned earlier, you will want to find a method of testing ketones in your body. One of the best ways to do this is to test your blood ketone levels using a meter. When you do this, the meter will be able to measure the amount of BHB in your blood, one of the primary ketones that will be present in your bloodstream. If you are in true Ketosis, your blood ketones should be anywhere from .5-3.0 mmol/L.

Weight Loss

When you first begin the ketogenic diet, weight loss can happen almost immediately. Some have reported that weight loss has even occurred in the first week! If this happens, the weight loss is most likely coming from the water and carbs that have been stored in your body.

Decreased Appetite

Another common symptom of the ketogenic diet is appetite suppression. Many individuals have reported that while following this diet, they aren't as hungry as they used to be. Potentially, this could be due to the increased protein intake and alterations to the hunger hormones through Ketosis. Either way, a decreased appetite means increased weight loss. It is a win-win situation for anyone following the ketogenic diet.

Increased Energy

When your body enters Ketosis, you will probably experience a new boost of energy that you didn't even know you had in you! Of course, increased energy and focus are a long-term effect of the diet. When you first start, you will most likely experience symptoms such as tiredness and brain fog. Fret not, as this is to be expected as your body adapts to a new fuel source.

The good news is that once you are in Ketosis, your brain is going to start burning these ketones instead of glucose. This is a very potent fuel for your mind, which is why followers of this diet have reported improved brain function and clarity.

Fatigue

As mentioned earlier, more than likely, you will experience some fatigue if you are just getting started on the ketogenic diet. On top of exhaustion, you may feel overall weak, which is a pretty common side effect of the ketogenic diet. As you probably realize, the switch to running on ketones isn't going to happen overnight. Instead, you should expect these symptoms to subside anywhere from seven to thirty days. To help combat the fatigue, consider taking an electrolyte supplement.

Digestive Issues

Another common symptom of starting this diet is experiencing digestive issues. When you make such a drastic change to your diet, it involves changing the types of foods you eat daily. When this happens, digestive problems like diarrhea and constipation are to be expected. While these symptoms will subside, you may want to take note of which foods you feel are causing these issues...

The Keto Flu and How to Survive

The ketogenic diet seems to be reasonably infamous for the keto flu. As your body begins to adapt to the new fuel source, it can genuinely feel like the flu. You may experience several symptoms such as dizziness, stomach pains, fatigue, and overall tiredness. For many beginners, this is the end of their attempt at the ketogenic diet.

You see, the keto flu is not caused by Ketosis or ketogenesis. The keto flu is caused by your body and its reaction to carbohydrate restriction! For many, this is the hardest part of following the ketogenic diet, but if you can make it through (I promise you can), incredible benefits are waiting on the other side.

The question here is, why is it so hard for the body to give up carbohydrates? You can look at carbs as your body's first love. Carbohydrates have provided free energy for your body up until this point. But, those carbohydrates are causing harm by increasing the risk of obesity, heart disease, and even diabetes. As you begin to break up with carbohydrates, it's going to be difficult at first.

While the adaption period is going to be difficult, through a proper diet of protein and fat, your body will begin to produce ketones and begin to feel so much better. But in the meantime, your body is going to have to adapt to different changes not just on a cellular level but also on a hormonal level. So, what can you expect when first starting? Below, you will find some of the signs and symptoms you are to expect in the first week or so of being the ketogenic diet.

Symptoms of the Keto Flu

While the keto flu may feel like the end of the world to some people, the good news is that it only lasts about a week for most people. You can expect these symptoms to begin around a day or two after you cut carbs from your diet. You can expect the following:

- Insomnia
- Confusion
- Muscle Soreness
- Nausea
- Stomach Pains
- Cramping
- Poor Concentration
- Irritability
- Inability to Focus
- Brain Fog
- Sugar Cravings
- Dizziness

Don't worry, though. You are likely experiencing only a few of these symptoms. For the lucky few, you may not even have gotten over the keto flu, but you better be prepared for the worst, just in case! You see, the keto flu affects everyone differently!

The main culprit for the keto flu will be your body's metabolic flexibility. This flexibility refers to its ability to adapt to the new availability and source of fuel. You may be wondering, can I be more flexible? The answer is yes, and no.

Your metabolic flexibility involves two things: genetics and lifestyle. If you look at it genetically, some people are born with less metabolic flexibility. For these unfortunate individuals, this means that it will be more challenging to adapt to the ketogenic diet, although not impossible.

If you want to be more flexible throughout your lifestyle, take a look at what you eat before starting the ketogenic diet. If your diet consists of a lot of processed foods and refined sugar, you are much more likely to experience the symptoms of a ketogenic diet.

Why Is This Happening to Me?

By having a deeper understanding of why keto flu occurs first, you will be able to understand better how to alleviate severe symptoms. Blessed with metabolic flexibility or not, your body undergoes drastic changes when you reduce carbohydrates. We've narrowed down some of the top culprits that can cause your symptoms.

Sodium and Water

First up, we have the fact that both water and sodium are now being flushed out of your system (bye water weight!) As you begin to restrict the number of carbohydrates in your diet, this is going to trigger the insulin release. As this insulin starts to tell your cells that there is an excess amount of energy in the body, this is going to make your kidneys to hold onto water and sodium. On the ketogenic diet, these levels are going to drop, and the sodium will be released from your body, taking all of the water with it. Typically, you can expect up to ten pounds of water weight lost in the first five days of your diet!

While seeing the number on your scale drop is going to be exciting, you will feel like garbage if this isn't taken care of properly. On top of the sodium and water leaving your body, the glycogen and fluid levels are going to be released as well. Through this process, the water loss could lead to symptoms such as headaches, dizziness, cramping, nausea, and gastrointestinal issues. This is why drinking the proper amount of water is going to be vital. You must replenish those minerals and fluids in your body.

Increased Cortisol Levels

As you begin the ketogenic diet, you will be triggering a response in your body, telling it that you are starving. While this is far from the truth, your body, who isn't used to living without carbohydrates, is going to release the stress hormone known as cortisol.

Once you become adapted to the ketones, these cortisol levels should balance out. Generally, this process takes a few weeks, depending on several different factors, including your diet, lifestyle, and that metabolic flexibility.

3. WHAT DOES THE KETOGENIC DIET MEAN FOR WOMEN AFTER 50?

Women who are looking for a quick and effective way to shed excess weight, get high blood sugar levels under control, reduce overall inflammations, and improve physical and mental energy will do their best by following a ketogenic diet plan. But there are special considerations women must take into account when they are beginning the keto diet.

All women know it is much more difficult for women to lose weight than it is for men to lose weight. A woman will live on a starvation level diet and exercise like a triathlete and only lose five pounds. A man will stop putting dressing on his salad and will lose twenty pounds. It just is not fair. But we have the fact that we are women to blame. Women naturally have more standing between them and weight loss than men do.

The mere fact that we are women is the largest single contributor to the reason we find it difficult to lose weight. Since our bodies always think they need to be prepared for the possibility of pregnancy women will naturally have more body fat and less mass in our muscles than men will. So, because we are women, we will always lose weight more slowly than men will.

Being in menopause will also cause women to add more pounds to their bodies, especially in the lower half of the body. After menopause, a woman's metabolism naturally slows down. Your hormone levels will decrease. These two factors alone will cause weight gain in the post-menopausal woman.

Women are a direct product of their hormones. Men also have hormones but not the ones like we have that regulate every function in our bodies. And the hormones in women will fluctuate around their everyday habits like lack of sleep, poor eating habits, and menstrual cycles. These hormones cause women to crave sweets around the time their periods occur. These cravings will wreck any diet plan. Staying true to the Keto plan is challenging at this time because of the intense desire for sweets and carbs. Also, having your period will often make you feel and look bloated because of the water your body holds onto during this time. And having cramps can make you more likely to reach for a bag of cookies than a plate of steak and salad.

Because we are women, we may experience challenges on the Keto diet that men will not face because they are men. One of these challenges is having a weight loss plateau or even experiencing weight gain. If this happens, you will want to increase your consumption of good fats like ghee, butter, eggs, coconut oil, beef, avocados, and olive oil. Any food that is cooked or prepared using oil must be prepared in olive oil or avocado oil.

You can also use MCT oil. MCT stands for medium-chain triglycerides. MCT can help with many body functions, from weight loss to improved brain function. MCTs are mostly missing from the typical American diet because we have been told that saturated fats are harmful to the body, and as a group they are. But certain saturated fats, like MCTs, are beneficial to the body, especially when they come from the right foods like beef or coconut oil.

Many women on a keto diet will struggle with imbalances in their hormones. On the keto diet, you do not rely on lowered calories to lose weight but on foods' effect on your hormones. So, when women begin the Keto diet, any issues they are already having with their hormones will be brought to attention and may cause the woman to give up before she starts. Always remember that the keto diet is responsible for cleansing the system first so that the body can quickly respond to the beautiful effects a keto diet has to offer.

Do not try to work toward the lean body that many men sport. It is best for an overall function that women stay at twenty-two to twenty-six percent body fat. Our hormones will function best in this range, and we can't possibly work without our hormones. Women who are very lean, like gymnasts and extreme athletes, will find their hormones no longer function or function at a less than optimal rate. And remember that ideal weight may not be the right weight for you. Many women find that they perform their best when they are at their happy weight. If you find yourself fighting with yourself to lose the last few pounds you think you need to lose to have the perfect body, then it may not be worth it. The struggle will affect your hormone function. Carefully observing the keto diet will allow time for your hormones to stabilize and regulate themselves back to their pre-obesity normal function.

Like any other diet plan, the keto diet will work better if you are active. Regular exercise will allow the body to strengthen and tone muscles and will help to work off excess fat reserves. But training requires energy to accomplish. If you restrict your carb intake too much, you might not have the energy needed to be physically able to make it through the day and still be able to maintain an exercise routine.

As a woman, you know that sometimes your emotions get the better of you. This is true with your body, as you well know, and can be a significant reason why women find it extremely difficult at times to lose weight the way they want to lose weight. We have been led to believe that not only can we do it all but that we must do it all. This gives many women extreme levels of pressure and can cause them to engage in emotional eating. Some women might have lowered feelings of self-worth and may not feel they are entitled to the benefits of the Keto diet, and turning to food relieves the feelings of inadequacy that we try to hide from the world.

When you engage in the same activity for an extended period, it becomes a habit. When you reach for the bag of potato chips or the tub of ice cream whenever you are angry, upset, or depressed, then your brain will eventually tell you to reach for food whenever you feel an emotion that you don't want to deal with. Food acts as a security blanket against the world outside. It may be necessary to address any extreme emotional issues you are having before you begin the Keto diet, so that you are better assured of success.

The actual act of staying on the Keto diet can be very challenging for some women. Many women see beginning a new diet to lose weight as a punishment for being overweight. It may be worthwhile for you to work at changing the settings of your mind if you are feeling this way. You may need to remind yourself daily that the Keto diet is not a punishment but a blessing for your body. Tell yourself that you do not deny yourself certain foods because you can't eat them, but because you do not like the way those foods make your body feel. Don't watch other people eating their high carb diet and pity yourself. Instead, feel sorry for the people who have trapped themselves in a high-calorie diet and are not experiencing the benefits that you are experiencing.

And for the first thirty days, cut out all sweeteners, even the non-sugar ones that are allowed on the Keto diet. While they may make food taste better, they also remind your brain that it needs sweet foods when it doesn't. Cutting them out for at least thirty days will break the cycle that your body has fallen into and will cut the cravings for sweets in your diet.

Women can be successful on the Keto diet if they are prepared to follow a few simple adjustments that will make the diet look differently than your male partner might be eating, but that will make you successful in the long run.

The third benefit from eating more fat, and perhaps the most important, is the psychological boost you will get from seeing that you can eat more fat and still lose weight and feel good. It will also reset your mindset that you formerly might have held against fat. For so long, we have been told that low fat is the only way to lose weight. But an absence of dietary fat will lead to overeating and binge eating out of a feeling of deprivation. When you begin the diet by allowing yourself to eat a lot, or too much in your mind, fat, then you swing the pendulum around to the other side of the fat scale where it properly belongs. You teach yourself that fat can be right for you. Increasing the extra intake of fats should not last beyond the second week of the diet. Your body will improve its ability to create and burn ketones and body fat, and then you will begin using your body fat for fuel, and you can begin to lower your reliance on dietary fat a little bit so that you will start to lose weight.

The Keto diet is naturally lower in calories if you follow the recommended levels of food intake. It is not necessary to try to restrict your intake of calories even further. All you need to do is to eat only until you are full and not one bite more. Besides losing weight, the Keto diet aims to retrain your body on how to work correctly. You will need to learn to trust your body and the signals it sends out to be able to readjust to a proper way of eating.

4. THE ULTIMATE KETO SHOPPING LIST

People complain about the difficulty of switching their shopping list to one that's Ketogenic-friendly. The fact is that food is expensive – and most of the food you have in your fridge is probably packed full of carbohydrates. If you're committing to a Ketogenic Diet, you need to do a clean sweep. That's right – everything that's packed with carbohydrates should be identified and set aside. You can donate them to a charity before going out and buying your new Keto-friendly shopping list.

Seafood

Seafood means fish like sardines, mackerel, and wild salmon. Go for shrimp, tuna, mussels, and crab into your diet. The secret is omega-3 fatty acids, which are credited for lots of health benefits. You want to add food rich in omega-3 fatty acids to your diet.

Low-Carb Vegetables

Not all vegetables are right for you when it comes to the Ketogenic Diet. The vegetable choices should be limited to those with low carbohydrate counts. Pack up your cart with items like spinach, eggplant, arugula, broccoli, and cauliflower. You can also put in bell peppers, cabbage, celery, kale, Brussels sprouts, mushrooms, zucchini, and fennel.

These vegetables also contain loads of fiber, which makes digestion easier. Of course, there's also the presence of vitamins, minerals, antioxidants, and various other nutrients that you need for day to day life.

Fruits Low in Sugar

During an episode of sugar-craving, it's usually a good idea to pick low-sugar fruit items. Just make sure to stock up on avocado, blackberries, raspberries, strawberries, blueberries, lime, lemon, and coconut. Also, note that tomatoes are fruits too, so feel free to make side dishes or dips with tomatoes' loads! Avocadoes are incredibly popular for those practicing the Ketogenic Diet because they contain LOTS of the right kind of fat.

Meat and Eggs

While some diets will tell you to skip the meat, the Ketogenic Diet encourages its consumption. Meat is packed with protein that will feed your muscles and give you a consistent energy source throughout the day. It's a slow but sure burn when you eat protein instead of carbohydrates, which are burned faster and therefore stored faster if you don't use them immediately.

But what kind of meat should you be eating? There's chicken, beef, pork, venison, turkey, and lamb. Keep in mind that quality plays a huge role here – you should be eating grass-fed organic beef or organic poultry if you want to make the most out of this food variety.

Nuts and Seeds

Nuts and seeds you should add to your cart include chia seeds, brazil nuts, macadamia nuts, flaxseed, walnuts, hemp seeds, pecans, sesame seeds, almonds, hazelnut, and pumpkin seeds. They also contain lots of protein and very little sugar, so they're great if you have an appetite. They're the ideal snack because they're quick, easy, and will keep you full. They're high in calories, though, which is why lots of people steer clear of them.

Dairy Products

OK – some people in their 50s already have a hard time processing dairy products, but you can happily add many of these to your diet for those who don't. Make sure to consume sufficient amounts of cheese, plain Greek yogurt, cream butter, and cottage cheese. These dairy products are packed with calcium, protein, and a healthy kind of fat.

Oils

Nope, we're not talking about essentials oils but rather MCT oil, coconut oil, avocado oil, nut oils, and even extra-virgin olive oil. You can start using those for your frying needs to create healthier food options. The beauty of these oils is that they add flavor to the food, making sure you don't get bored quickly with the recipes. Try picking up different types of Keto-friendly oils to add some variety to your cooking.

Coffee and Tea

Instead, beverages would be limited to unsweetened tea or unsweetened coffee to keep sugar consumption low. Opt for organic coffee and tea products to make the most out of these powerful antioxidants.

Dark Chocolate

Yes – chocolate is still on the menu, but it is limited to just dark chocolate. Technically, this means eating chocolate that is 70 percent cacao, which would make the taste a bit bitter.

Sugar Substitutes

In a while, the part of this book's recipe, you might be surprised at some of the ingredients required in the list. Because while sweeteners are an essential part of food preparation, you can't just use any sugar in your recipe. Remember: the regular sugar is pure carbohydrate. Even if you're not eating carbohydrates, if you're dumping lots of sugar in your food – you're not following the Ketogenic Diet principles.

So, what do you do? You find sugar substitutes. You can get rid of the old sugar and use any of these as a good substitute.

- Stevia. Perhaps the most familiar one in this list. It's a natural sweetener derived from plants and contains very few calories. Typically, the ratio is 200 grams of sugar per 1 teaspoon of powdered stevia.

- Sucralose. It contains zero calories and zero carbohydrates. It's an artificial sweetener and does not metabolize – hence the complete lack of carbohydrates.

- Erythritol. It's a naturally occurring compound that interacts with the tongue's sweet taste receptors. Hence, it mimics the taste of sugar without actually being sugar. It does contain calories, but only about 5% of the calories you'll find in the regular sugar.

- Xylitol. It still contains calories; the calories are just 3 per gram. It's a sweetener that's good for diabetic patients because it doesn't raise the body's sugar levels.

What About Condiments?

Condiments are still on the table, but they won't be as tasty as you're used to. Your options include mustard, olive oil mayonnaise, oil-based salad dressings, and unsweetened ketchup. Of all these condiments, ketchup is the one with the most sugar, so make a point of looking for one with reduced sugar content.

What About Snacks?

The good news is that there are packed snacks for those who don't have the time to make it themselves. Sugarless nut butter, dried seaweeds, nuts, and sugar-free jerky are all available in stores.

Once you've figured this out, you can quickly make calculations in your head about the carbohydrate content of what you're eating based on the labels. You will find that this can be easily adjusted to your eating habits so that you always know what you're consuming, even if you're not following a set recipe.

5. MENOPAUSE AND THE KETOGENIC DIET

For aging women, menopause will bring severe changes and challenges, but a ketogenic diet can help you effortlessly switch gears to continue enjoying a healthy and happy life. Menopause can alter hormone levels in women, which in turn affects the brain's ability and cognitive abilities. Also, due to the lower production of estrogen and progesterone, your sex drive is lowered, and you suffer from sleep and mood problems. Let's take a look at how a ketogenic diet will help resolve these side effects.

Enhanced Cognitive Functions

Usually, the hormone estrogen ensures a constant flow of glucose to your brain. But after menopause, estrogen levels begin to drop dramatically, as does the amount of glucose in bran. As a result, the available power of your brain will start to deteriorate. However, by following the ketogenic diet for women over 50, the problem of glucose intake is avoided. This results in improved cognitive functions and brain activity.

Hormonal Balance

Usually, women experience significant menopausal symptoms due to hormonal imbalances. The ketogenic diet for women over 50 works by stabilizing these imbalances like estrogen. This helps show tolerable minor menopausal symptoms, such as hot flashes. The keto diet also balances insulin and blood sugar levels and helps control insulin sensitivity.

Intense Sex Drive

The ketogenic diet increases the absorption of vitamin D, which is essential for improving sexual desire. Vitamin D ensures stable levels of testosterone and other sex hormones that could become unstable due to low testosterone levels.

Better Sleep

Glucose alters your blood sugar levels, which in turn leads to a low quality of sleep. Along with other symptoms of menopause, sleeping well becomes a big problem as you age. The ketogenic diet for women over 50 not only balances blood glucose levels, but also stabilizes other hormones such as cortisol, melatonin, and serotonin that ensure better and better sleep.

Reduces Inflammation

Menopause can increase inflammation levels by leaving potentially harmful invaders in our system, resulting in unpleasant and painful symptoms. The ketogenic diet for women over 50 uses healthy anti-inflammatory fats to reduce inflammation and pain in the joints and bones.

Fill Your Brain

Did you know that your brain is made up of 60% fat or more? This means that more fat is needed to maintain optimal function. In other words, the ketones in the ketogenic diet serve as an energy source that fuels brain cells.

Nutrient Deficiencies

Aging women tend to have more significant deficiencies in essential nutrients such as iron deficiency, leading to mental confusion and fatigue. Vitamin B12 deficiency, leading to neurological conditions such as dementia. Fat lack, which can cause problems with knowledge, skin, vision, and vitamin D deficiency that not only causes cognitive decline in older adults and increases the risk of heart disease but also contributes to the risk of developing cancer. On a ketogenic diet, high-quality protein provides excellent and adequate sources of these essential nutrients.

6. BREAKFAST

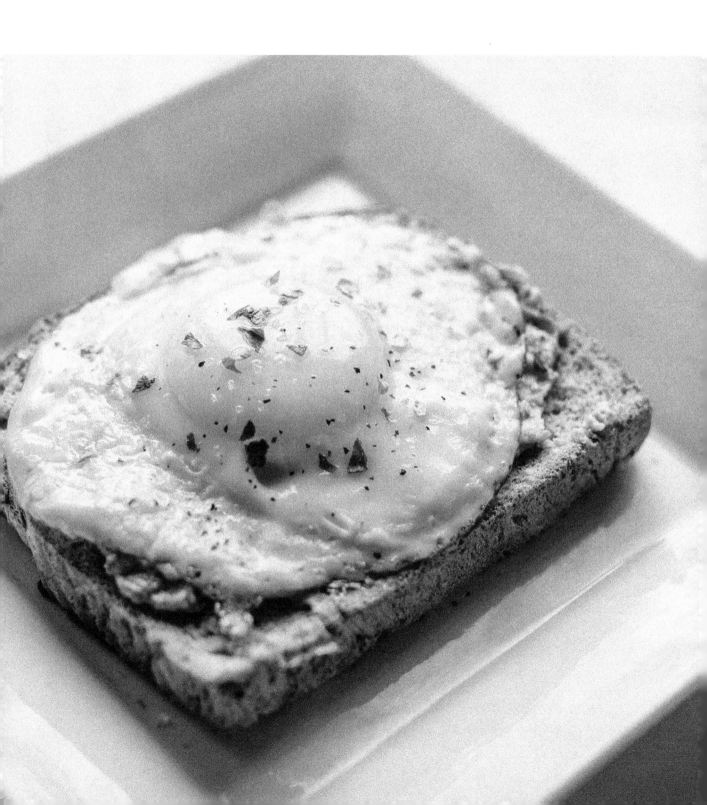

PREPARATION: 15 MIN **COOKING: 20 MIN** **SERVES: 4**

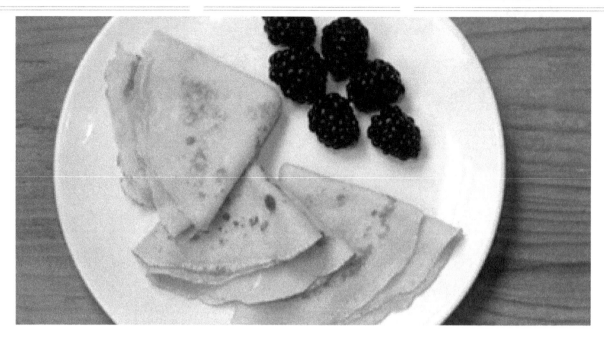

CHEESE CREPES

INGREDIENTS

- 6 ounces cream cheese, softened
- 1/3 cup Parmesan cheese, grated
- 6 large organic eggs
- 1 teaspoon granulated erythritol
- 1½ tablespoon coconut flour
- 1/8 teaspoon xanthan gum
- 2 tablespoons unsalted butter

DIRECTIONS

1. In a blender, add cream cheese, Parmesan cheese, eggs, and erythritol, and pulse on low speed until well combined.
2. While the motor is running, place the coconut flour and xanthan gum and pulse until a thick mixture is formed.
3. Now, pulse on medium speed for a few seconds.
4. Transfer the mixture into a bowl and set aside for about 5 minutes.
5. Divide the mixture into 10 equal-sized portions.
6. In a nonstick pan, melt butter over medium-low heat.
7. Place 1 portion of the mixture and tilt the pan to spread into a thin layer.
8. Cook for about 1½ minutes or until the edges become brown.
9. Flip the crepe and cook for about 15-20 seconds more.
10. Repeat with the remaining mixture.
11. Serve warm with your favorite keto-friendly filling.

Nutritions: *Calories 297 Net Carbs 1.9 g Total Carbs 3.5 Fiber 1.6 g Sugar 0.5 g Protein 13.7 g*

PREPARATION: 10 MIN **COOKING: 20 MIN** **SERVES: 5**

RICOTTA PANCAKES

INGREDIENTS

- 4 organic eggs
- ½ cup ricotta cheese
- ¼ cup unsweetened vanilla whey protein powder
- ½ teaspoon organic baking powder
- Pinch of salt
- ½ teaspoon liquid stevia
- 2 tablespoons unsalted butter

DIRECTIONS

1. In a blender, add all the ingredients and pulse until well combined.
2. In a wok, melt butter over medium heat.
3. Add the desired amount of the mixture and spread it evenly.
4. Cook for about 2–3 minutes or until the bottom becomes golden-brown.
5. Flip and cook for about 1–2 minutes or until golden brown.
6. Repeat with the remaining mixture.
7. Serve warm.

Nutritions: *Calories 184 Net Carbs 2.7 g Total Carbs 2.7 g Fiber 0 Sugar 0.8 g Protein 14.6 g*

PREPARATION: 15 MIN **COOKING: 25 MIN** **SERVES: 4**

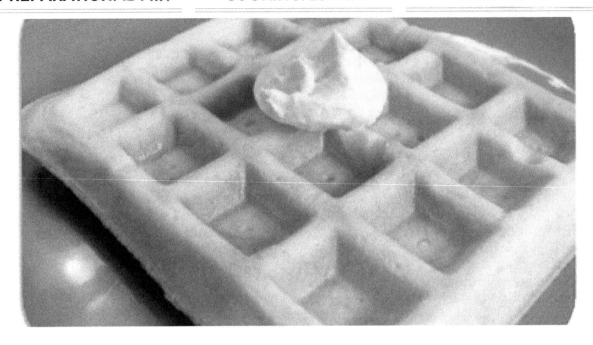

YOGURT WAFFLES

INGREDIENTS

- ½ cup golden flax seeds meal
- ½ cup plus 3 tablespoons almond flour
- 1-1½ tablespoons granulated erythritol
- 1 tablespoon unsweetened vanilla whey protein powder
- ½ teaspoon organic powder
- ¼ teaspoon xanthan gum
- Salt, as required
- 1 large organic egg, white and yolk separated
- 1 organic whole egg
- 2 tablespoons unsweetened almond milk
- 1½ tablespoons unsalted butter
- 3 ounces plain Greek yogurt
- ¼ teaspoon baking soda

DIRECTIONS

1. Preheat the waffle iron and then grease it.
2. In a large bowl, add the flour, erythritol, protein powder, baking soda, baking powder, xanthan gum, and salt, and mix until well combined.
3. In a second small bowl, add the egg white and beat until stiff peaks form.
4. In a third bowl, add 2 egg yolks, whole egg, almond milk, butter, and yogurt, and beat until well combined.
5. Place egg mixture into the bowl of flour mixture and mix until well combined.
6. Gently, fold in the beaten egg whites.
7. Place ¼ cup of the mixture into preheated waffle iron and cook for about 4–5 minutes or until golden brown.
8. Repeat with the remaining mixture.
9. Serve warm.

Nutritions: *Calories 250 Net Carbs 3.2 g Total Carbs 8.8 g Fiber 5.6 g Sugar 1.3 g Protein 8.4 g*

PREPARATION: 15 MIN   **COOKING: 20 MIN**   **SERVES: 5**

BROCCOLI MUFFINS

INGREDIENTS

- 2 tablespoons unsalted butter
- 6 large organic eggs
- ½ cup heavy whipping cream
- ½ cup Parmesan cheese, grated
- Salt and ground black pepper, as required
- 1¼ cups broccoli, chopped
- 2 tablespoons fresh parsley, chopped
- ½ cup Swiss cheese, grated

DIRECTIONS

1. Preheat your oven to 350°F.
2. Grease a 12-cup muffin tin.
3. In a bowl, add the eggs, cream, Parmesan cheese, salt, and black pepper, and beat until well combined.
4. Divide the broccoli and parsley in the bottom of each prepared muffin cup evenly.
5. Top with the egg mixture, followed by the Swiss cheese.
6. Bake for about 20 minutes, rotating the pan once halfway through.
7. Remove from the oven and place onto a wire rack for about 5 minutes before serving.
8. Carefully, invert the muffins onto a serving platter and serve warm.

Nutritions: *Calories 231 Net Carbs 2 g Total Carbs 2.5 g Fiber 0.5 g Sugar 0.9 g Protein 13.5 g*

PREPARATION: 15 MIN **COOKING: 1 HOUR** **SERVES: 5**

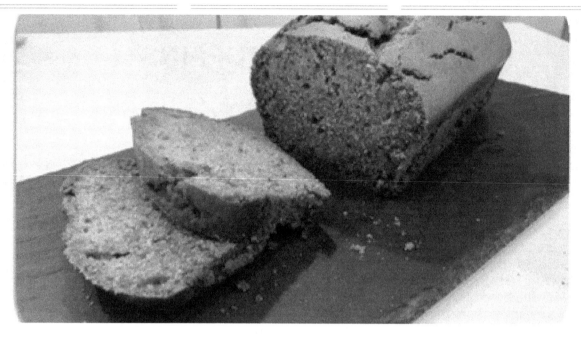

PUMPKIN BREAD

INGREDIENTS

- 1 2/3 cups almond flour
- 1½ teaspoons organic baking powder
- ½ teaspoon pumpkin pie spice
- ½ teaspoon ground cinnamon
- ½ teaspoon ground cloves
- ½ teaspoon salt
- 8 ounces cream cheese, softened
- 6 organic eggs, divided
- 1 tablespoon coconut flour
- 1 cup powdered erythritol, divided
- 1 teaspoon stevia powder, divided
- 1 teaspoon organic lemon extract
- 1 cup homemade pumpkin puree
- ½ cup coconut oil, melted

DIRECTIONS

1. Preheat your oven to 325°F.
2. Lightly grease 2 bread loaf pans.
3. In a bowl, place almond flour, baking powder, spices, and salt, and mix until well combined.
4. In a second bowl, add the cream cheese, 1 egg, coconut flour, ¼ cup of erythritol, and ¼ teaspoon of the stevia, and with a wire whisk, beat until smooth.
5. In a third bowl, add the pumpkin puree, oil, 5 eggs, ¾ cup of the erythritol, and ¾ teaspoon of the stevia, and with a wire whisk, beat until well combined.
6. Add the pumpkin mixture into the bowl of the flour mixture and mix until just combined.
7. Place about ¼ of the pumpkin mixture into each loaf pan evenly.
8. Top each pan with the cream cheese mixture evenly, followed by the remaining pumpkin mixture.
9. Bake for about 50–60 minutes or until a toothpick inserted in the center comes out clean.
10. Remove the bread pans from the oven and place onto a wire rack, and let it be for 10 minutes.
11. With a sharp knife, cut each bread loaf into the desired-sized slices and serve.

Nutritions: *Calories 216 Net Carbs 2.5 g Total Carbs 4.5 g Fiber 2 g Sugar 1.1 g Protein 3.4 g*

PREPARATION: 10 MIN **COOKING: 20 MIN** **SERVES: 4**

EGGS IN AVOCADO CUPS

INGREDIENTS

- 2 ripe avocados, halved and pitted
- 4 organic eggs
- Salt and ground black pepper, as required
- 4 tablespoons cheddar cheese, shredded
- 2 cooked bacon slices, chopped
- 1 tablespoon scallion greens, chopped

DIRECTIONS

1. Preheat your oven to 400°F.
2. Carefully remove abut about 2 tablespoons of flesh from each avocado half.
3. Place avocado halves into a small baking dish.
4. Carefully crack an egg in each avocado half and sprinkle with salt and black pepper.
5. Top each egg with cheddar cheese evenly.
6. Bake for about 20 minutes or until the desired doneness of the eggs.
7. Serve immediately with the garnishing of bacon and chives.

Nutritions: *Calories 343 Net Carbs 2.2 g Total Carbs 7.9 g Fiber 5.7 g Sugar 0.8 g Protein 13.8 g*

PREPARATION: 10 MIN **COOKING: 8 MIN** **SERVES: 2**

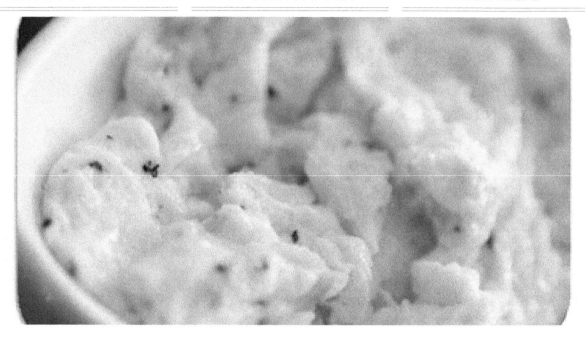

CHEDDAR SCRAMBLE

INGREDIENTS

- 2 tablespoons olive oil
- 1 small yellow onion, chopped finely
- 12 large organic eggs, beaten lightly
- Salt and ground black pepper, as required
- 4 ounces cheddar cheese, shredded

DIRECTIONS

1. In a large wok, heat oil over medium heat and sauté the onion for about 4–5 minutes.
2. Add the eggs, salt, and black pepper and cook for about 3 minutes, stirring continuously.
3. Remove from the heat and immediately stir in the cheese.
4. Serve immediately.

Nutritions: *Calories 264 Net Carbs 1.8 g Total Carbs 2.1 g Fiber 0.3 g Sugar 1.4 g Protein 17.4 g*

PREPARATION: 10 MIN **COOKING: 15 MIN** **SERVES: 3**

BACON OMELET

INGREDIENTS

- 4 large organic eggs
- 1 tablespoon fresh chives, minced
- Salt and ground black pepper, as required
- 4 bacon slices
- 1 tablespoon unsalted butter
- 2 ounces cheddar cheese, shredded

DIRECTIONS

1. In a bowl, add the eggs, chives, salt, and black pepper, and beat until well combined.
2. Heat a non-stick frying pan over medium-high heat and cook the bacon slices for about 8–10 minutes.
3. Place the bacon onto a paper towel-lined plate to drain. Then chop the bacon slices.
4. With paper towels, wipe out the frying pan.
5. In the same frying pan, melt butter over medium-low heat and cook the egg mixture for about 2 minutes.
6. Carefully, flip the omelet and top with chopped bacon.
7. Cook for 1–2 minutes or until desired doneness of eggs.
8. Remove from heat and immediately, place the cheese in the center of omelet.
9. Fold the edges of omelet over cheese and cut into 2 portions.
10. Serve immediately.

Nutritions: *Calories 427 Net Carbs 1.2 g Total Carbs 1.2 g Fiber 0 g Sugar 1 g Protein 29.1 g*

PREPARATION: 20 MIN **COOKING: 20 MIN** **SERVES: 5**

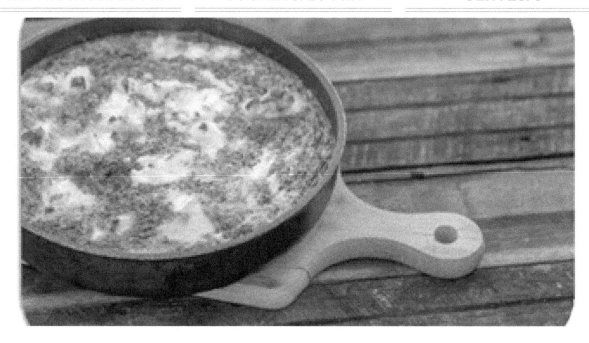

GREEN VEGGIES QUICHE

INGREDIENTS

- 6 organic eggs
- ½ cup unsweetened almond milk
- Salt and ground black pepper, as required
- 2 cups fresh baby spinach, chopped
- ½ cup green bell pepper, seeded and chopped
- 1 scallion, chopped
- ¼ cup fresh cilantro, chopped
- 1 tablespoon fresh chives, minced
- 3 tablespoons mozzarella cheese, grated

DIRECTIONS

1. Preheat your oven to 400°F.
2. Lightly grease a pie dish.
3. In a bowl, add eggs, almond milk, salt, and black pepper, and beat until well combined. Set aside.
4. In another bowl, add the vegetables and herbs and mix well.
5. In the bottom of the prepared pie dish, place the veggie mixture evenly and top with the egg mixture.
6. Bake for about 20 minutes or until a wooden skewer inserted in the center comes out clean.
7. Remove pie dish from the oven and immediately sprinkle with the Parmesan cheese.
8. Set aside for about 5 minutes before slicing.
9. Cut into desired sized wedges and serve warm.

Nutritions: *Calories 176 Net Carbs 4.1 g Total Carbs 5 g Fiber 0.9 g Sugar 4 g Protein 15.4 g*

PREPARATION: 15 MIN **COOKING: 12 MIN** **SERVES: 4**

CHICKEN & ASPARAGUS FRITTATA

INGREDIENTS

- ½ cup grass-fed cooked chicken breast, chopped
- 1/3 cup Parmesan cheese, grated
- 6 organic eggs, beaten lightly
- Salt and ground black pepper, as required
- 1/3 cup boiled asparagus, chopped
- ¼ cup cherry tomatoes, halved
- ¼ cup mozzarella cheese, shredded

DIRECTIONS

1. Preheat the broiler of the oven.
2. In a bowl, add the Parmesan cheese, eggs, salt, and black pepper, and beat until well combined.
3. In a large ovenproof wok, melt butter over medium-high heat and cook the chicken and asparagus for about 2–3 minutes.
4. Add the egg mixture and tomatoes and stir to combine.
5. Cook for about 4–5 minutes.
6. Remove from the heat and sprinkle with the Parmesan cheese.
7. Now, transfer the wok under the broiler and broil for about 3–4 minutes or until slightly puffed.
8. Cut into desired sized wedges and serve immediately.

Nutritions: *Calories 158 Net Carbs 1.3 g Total Carbs 1.7 g Fiber 0.4 g Sugar 1 g*

7. LUNCH

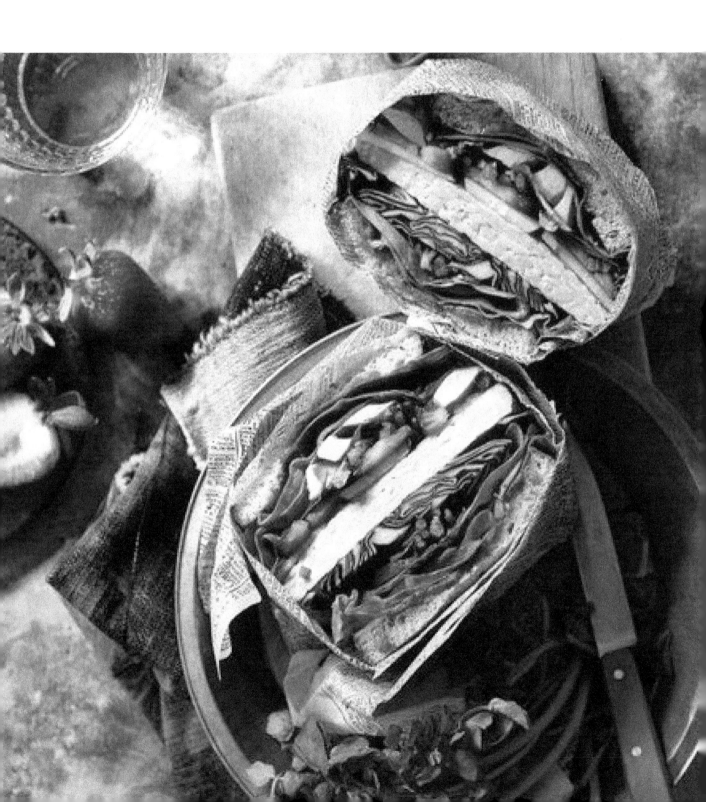

PREPARATION: 12 MIN **COOKING: 15 MIN** **SERVES: 20**

KETO BURGER FAT BOMBS

INGREDIENTS

- Cooking spray
- 1 lb. ground beef
- 1/2 tsp. garlic powder
- Kosher salt
- Freshly ground black pepper
- 2 tbsp. cold butter, cut into 20 pieces
- 2 oz. cheddar, cut into 20 pieces
- Lettuce leaves, for serving
- Thinly sliced tomatoes, for serving
- Mustard, for serving

DIRECTIONS

1. Heat oven to 375 °F (190 °C), grease a mini muffin tin with cooking spray.
2. In a medium bowl, season beef with garlic powder, salt, and pepper.
3. Press one teaspoon beef consistently into the bottom of each muffin tin cup, totally covering the bottom.
4. Place a slice of butter on top, then press one teaspoon beef over butter to cover.
5. Place a slice of cheddar on top of meat in each cup, then press remaining beef over cheese to cover.
6. Bake the fat bombs until the meat is golden and cook through for about 15 minutes.
7. Let cool slightly.
8. Carefully use a metal offset spatula to release each burger from the tin. Serve with lettuce leaves, tomatoes, and mustard.
9. Enjoy!

Nutritions: *Calories: 77.5 Carbohydrates: 1.7g Fat: 4.8g Protein: 6.3g*

PREPARATION: 12 MIN **COOKING: 20 MIN** **SERVES: 12**

KETO TACO CUPS

INGREDIENTS

- 2 c. Shredded cheddar
- 1 tbsp. Extra-virgin olive oil
- 1 small onion, chopped
- 3 cloves garlic, minced
- 1 lb. Ground beef
- 1 tsp. Chili powder
- 1/2 tsp. Ground cumin
- 1/2 Tsp. Paprika
- Kosher salt
- Freshly ground black pepper
- Sour cream, for serving
- Diced avocado, for serving
- Freshly chopped cilantro, for serving
- Chopped tomatoes, for serving

DIRECTIONS

1. Preheat oven to 375 °F (190 °C).
2. Line a large baking tray with parchment paper or a baking mat.
3. Put about 2 tablespoons cheddar with a space of 2-inches.
4. Bake the cheese until bubbly and edges turn to golden, about 5-7 minutes.
5. Let the crisps cool on the baking sheet for a minute.
6. Grease the bottom of a muffin tin with cooking spray set aside.
7. Put the backed melted cheese slices on the bottom of a muffin tin.
8. Top with another muffin tin and let it cool for 8-10 minutes.
9. Heat oil in a skillet over medium heat, add chopped onion, and cook until soft.
10. Add garlic and cook until fragrant, add ground beef, breaking up meat with a spatula.
11. Cook until the beef is browned and no longer pink, about 4-6 minutes, then drain the fat.
12. Add the meat again to the skillet and season with chili powder, cumin, paprika, salt, and pepper.
13. Place cheese cups on a serving platter.
14. Fill the cheese cups with cooked ground beef and top with sour cream, avocado, cilantro, and tomatoes.
15. Enjoy!

Nutritions: *Calories: 189.8 Carbohydrates: 1.1g Fat: 14.2g Protein: 14.2g*

PREPARATION: 25 MIN **COOKING: 0 MIN** **SERVES: 4**

CAPRESE ZOODLES

INGREDIENTS

- 4 large zucchini
- 2 tbsp. Extra-virgin olive oil
- Kosher salt
- Freshly ground black pepper
- 2 c. Cherry tomatoes halved
- 1 c. Mozzarella balls, quartered if large
- 1/4 c. Fresh basil leaves
- 2 tbsp. Balsamic vinegar

DIRECTIONS

1. Using a spiralizer, make zoodles out of zucchini.
2. Put zoodles in a big bowl, toss with olive oil, and season with pepper and salt.
3. Let marinate for 15 minutes.
4. Combine with tomatoes, mozzarella, and basil to zoodles in a bowl and toss until combined.
5. Drizzle with balsamic and serve.
6. Enjoy!

Nutritions: *Calories: 311 Carbohydrates: 7.4g Fat: 22.2g Protein:16.7g*

PREPARATION: 20 MIN **COOKING: 0 MIN** **SERVES: 2**

ZUCCHINI SUSHI

INGREDIENTS

- 2 medium zucchini
- 4 oz. cream cheese softened
- 1 tsp. Sriracha hot sauce
- 1 tsp. lime juice
- 1 c. lump crab meat
- 1/2 carrot, cut into thin matchsticks
- 1/2 avocado, diced
- 1/2 cucumber, cut into thin matchsticks
- 1 tsp. toasted sesame seeds

DIRECTIONS

1. With a vegetable peeler, slice each zucchini into even thin strips.
2. Place zucchini on a lined plate to dry up the moisture.
3. In a bowl, whisk together cream cheese, Sriracha, and lime juice.
4. Place two zucchini slices down straight on a cutting board.
5. Top with cream cheese in a thin layer on the lift side top with crab, cucumber, and avocado.
6. Roll the zucchini tightly from the lift side.
7. Repeat the process with the remaining zucchini pieces.
8. Garnish with sesame seeds before serving.

Nutritions: *Calories: 378.8 Carbohydrates: 10.5g Fat: 25.5g Protein: 27.7g*

PREPARATION: 13 MIN **COOKING: 15 MIN** **SERVES: 4**

ASIAN CHICKEN LETTUCE WRAPS

INGREDIENTS

- 3 tbsp. hoisin sauce
- 2 tbsp. low-sodium soy sauce
- 2 tbsp. rice wine vinegar
- 1 tbsp. Sriracha (optional)
- 1 tsp. sesame oil
- 1 tbsp. extra-virgin olive oil
- 1 medium onion, diced
- 2 cloves garlic, minced
- 1 tbsp. freshly grated ginger
- 1 lb. ground chicken
- 1/2 c. water chestnuts, drained and sliced
- 2 green onions, thinly sliced
- Kosher salt
- Freshly ground black pepper
- Large leafy lettuce (leaves separated), for serving

DIRECTIONS

1. Whisk together hoisin sauce, rice wine vinegar, soy sauce, Sriracha, and sesame oil in a bowl.
2. In a big skillet over medium-high heat, preheat olive oil.
3. Put onions and cook until soft, about 5 minutes.
4. Then stir in garlic and ginger and cook until fragrant, about 1 minute more.
5. Put ground chicken and cook until opaque and typically cooked through, breaking up meat with a wooden spoon.
6. Pour in the sauce and cook 1 to 2 minutes more, until sauce reduces slightly and chicken cooked through thoroughly.
7. Turn off heat and stir in chestnuts and green onions.
8. Season with pepper and salt.
9. Spoon rice, if using, and a large scoop (about 1/4 cup) of chicken mixture into the center of each lettuce leaf. Serve immediately.

Nutritions: *Calories: 280.85 Carbohydrates: 8.7g Fat: 17.6g Protein: 21.4g*

PREPARATION: 11 MIN **COOKING: 15 MIN** **SERVES: 4**

PROSCIUTTO AND MOZZARELLA BOMB

INGREDIENTS

- 4 oz (113g) sliced prosciutto
- 8 oz (226g) fresh mozzarella ball
- Olive oil, for frying

DIRECTIONS

1. Coating half of the prosciutto slices vertically.
2. Lay the remaining slices horizontally across the first set of slices.
3. Place your mozzarella ball, upside down, onto the crisscrossed prosciutto slices.
4. Firmly, but very carefully, wrap the mozzarella ball with the prosciutto slices.
5. If making ahead, wrap the balls in cling film and refrigerate.
6. To serve, heat the olive oil in a skillet and crisp the prosciutto on all sides.
7. Enjoy!

Nutritions: *Calories: 129 Carbohydrates: 0.3g Fat: 11.6g Protein: 6.2g*

PREPARATION: 14 MIN **COOKING: 21 MIN** **SERVES: 8**

KETOFIED CHICK-FIL-A-STYLE CHICKEN

INGREDIENTS

- 24-oz (680g) pickle jar
- 8 medium uncooked chicken breast tenders
- 4 tbsp. almond flour
- ¼ cup grated Parmesan
- Salt and pepper, to taste
- 1 tsp. paprika
- 2 large eggs
- 2 tbsp. avocado oil

DIRECTIONS

1. In a plastic resealable bag, add the chicken and the pickle juice, marinate in the fridge for 20-30 minutes.
2. On a plate, combine the almond flour, grated Parmesan, salt, pepper, and paprika.
3. Whip the eggs together in a separate bowl.
4. Preheat a skillet over medium-high heat and heat the avocado oil.
5. First, dip the chicken pieces in the beaten egg, then place it in the breading mixture to coat.
6. Place the chicken into the skillet and cook until golden browned.

Nutritions: *Calories: 407 Carbohydrates: 12.5g Fat: 23.6g Protein: 28g*

PREPARATION: 7 MIN   **COOKING: 25 MIN**   **SERVES: 4**

CHEESEBURGER TOMATOES

INGREDIENTS

- 1 tbsp. extra-virgin olive oil
- 1 medium onion, chopped
- 2 cloves garlic, minced
- 1 lb. ground beef
- 1 tbsp. ketchup
- 1 tbsp. yellow mustard
- 4 slicing tomatoes
- Kosher salt
- Freshly ground black pepper
- 2/3 c. shredded cheddar
- 1/4 c. shredded iceberg lettuce
- 4 pickle coins
- Sesame seeds, for garnish

DIRECTIONS

1. In a skillet over medium heat, heat oil.
2. Put onion and cook until tender, about 5 minutes, then stir in garlic.
3. Place ground beef, cook and break up the meat with a spatula, cook until the beef browned about 6 minutes, drain fat.
4. Season with salt and pepper, then add the ketchup and mustard.
5. Flip tomatoes so they are stem-side down.
6. Cut the tomatoes into six wedges, being careful not to cut entirely through the tomatoes.
7. Carefully spread open the wedges.
8. Divide cooked ground beef evenly among the tomatoes.
9. Then top each with cheese and lettuce.
10. Garnish with pickle coins and sesame seeds.
11. Serve it and enjoy it!

Nutritions: *Calories: 458 Carbohydrates: 5g Fat: 32.8g Protein: 33.4g*

8. DINNER

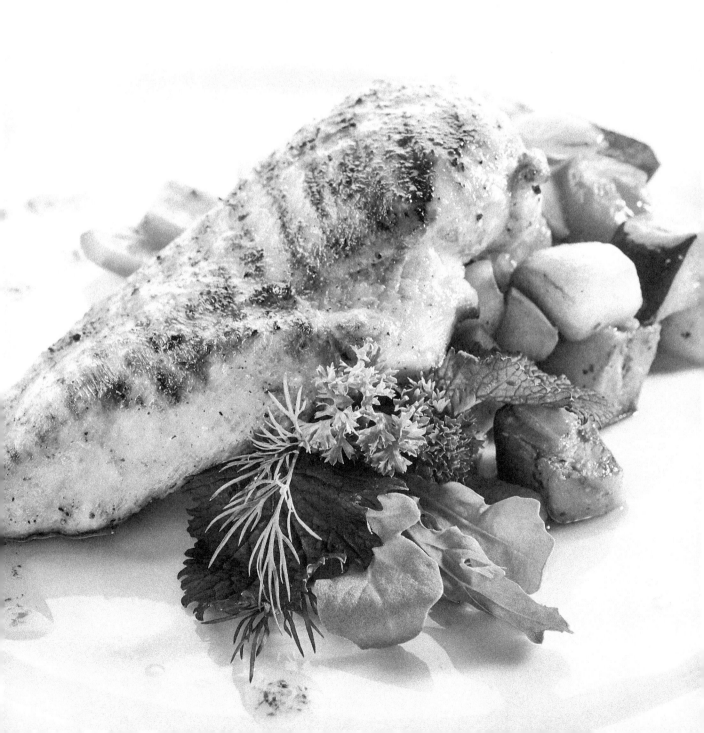

PREPARATION: 10 MIN   **COOKING: 25 MIN**   **SERVES: 6**

KORMA CURRY

INGREDIENTS

- 3-pound chicken breast, skinless, boneless
- 1 teaspoon garam masala
- 1 teaspoon curry powder
- 1 tablespoon apple cider vinegar
- ½ coconut cream
- 1 cup organic almond milk
- 1 teaspoon ground coriander
- ¾ teaspoon ground cardamom
- ½ teaspoon ginger powder
- ¼ teaspoon cayenne pepper
- ¾ teaspoon ground cinnamon
- 1 tomato, diced
- 1 teaspoon avocado oil
- ½ cup of water

DIRECTIONS

1. Chop the chicken breast and put it in the saucepan.
2. Add avocado oil and start to cook it over medium heat.
3. Sprinkle the chicken with garam masala, curry powder, apple cider vinegar, ground coriander, cardamom, ginger powder, cayenne pepper, ground cinnamon, and diced tomato. Mix up the ingredients carefully. Cook them for 10 minutes.
4. Add water, coconut cream, and almond milk. Saute the meat for 10 minutes more.

Nutritions: *Calories: 440 Fat: 32g Fiber: 4g Carbohydrates: 28g Protein: 8g*

PREPARATION: 10 MIN **COOKING: 15 MIN** **SERVES: 8**

ZUCCHINI BARS

INGREDIENTS

- 3 zucchini, grated
- ½ white onion, diced
- 2 teaspoons butter
- 3 eggs, whisked
- 4 tablespoons coconut flour
- 1 teaspoon salt
- ½ teaspoon ground black pepper
- 5 oz goat cheese, crumbled
- 4 oz Swiss cheese, shredded
- ½ cup spinach, chopped
- 1 teaspoon baking powder
- ½ teaspoon lemon juice

DIRECTIONS

1. In the mixing bowl, mix up together grated zucchini, diced onion, eggs, coconut flour, salt, ground black pepper, crumbled cheese, chopped spinach, baking powder, and lemon juice.
2. Add butter and churn the mixture until homogenous.
3. Line the baking dish with baking paper.
4. Transfer the zucchini mixture into the baking dish and flatten it.
5. Preheat the oven to 365F and put the dish inside.
6. Cook it for 15 minutes. Then chill the meal well.
7. Cut it into bars.

Nutritions: *Calories: 187.2 Total Fat: 7.3 g Saturated Fat: 0.6 g Cholesterol: 17.6 mg Sodium: 29.5 mg Potassium: 74.2 mg Total Carbohydrate: 29.5 g Protein: 1.7 g*

PREPARATION: 10 MIN **COOKING: 25 MIN** **SERVES: 4**

MUSHROOM SOUP

INGREDIENTS

- 1 cup of water
- 1 cup of coconut milk
- 1 cup white mushrooms, chopped
- ½ carrot, chopped
- ¼ white onion, diced
- 1 tablespoon butter
- 2 oz turnip, chopped
- 1 teaspoon dried dill
- ½ teaspoon ground black pepper
- ¾ teaspoon smoked paprika
- 1 oz celery stalk, chopped

DIRECTIONS

1. Pour water and coconut milk into the saucepan. Bring the liquid to a boil.
2. Add chopped mushrooms, carrots, and turnips. Close the lid and boil for 10 minutes.
3. Meanwhile, put butter in the skillet. Add diced onion. Sprinkle it with dill, ground black pepper, and smoked paprika. Roast the onion for 3 minutes.
4. Add the roasted onion to the soup mixture.
5. Then add chopped celery stalk. Close the lid.
6. Cook soup for 10 minutes.
7. Then ladle it into the serving bowls.

Nutritions: *Calories: 39 Total Fat: 2.6 g Cholesterol: 0 mg Sodium: 340 mg Potassium: 31 mg Total Carbohydrate: 3.3 g Protein: 0.7 g*

PREPARATION: 10 MIN   **COOKING: 10 MIN**   **SERVES: 4**

STUFFED PORTOBELLO MUSHROOMS

INGREDIENTS

- 2 portobello mushrooms
- 1 cup spinach, chopped, steamed
- 2 oz artichoke hearts, drained, chopped
- 1 tablespoon coconut cream
- 1 tablespoon cream cheese
- 1 teaspoon minced garlic
- 1 tablespoon fresh cilantro, chopped
- 3 oz Cheddar cheese, grated
- ½ teaspoon ground black pepper
- 2 tablespoons olive oil
- ½ teaspoon salt

DIRECTIONS

1. Sprinkle mushrooms with olive oil and place them in the tray.
2. Transfer the tray to the preheated to 360F oven and broil them for 5 minutes.
3. Meanwhile, blend artichoke hearts, coconut cream, cream cheese, minced garlic, and chopped cilantro.
4. Add grated cheese to the mixture and sprinkle with ground black pepper and salt.
5. Fill the broiled mushrooms with the cheese mixture and cook them for 5 minutes more. Serve the mushrooms only hot.

Nutritions: *Calories: 135.2 Total Fat: 5.5 g Cholesterol: 16.4 mg Sodium: 698.1 mg Potassium: 275.3 mg Total Carbohydrate: 8.4 g Protein: 14.8 g*

PREPARATION: 10 MIN **COOKING: /** **SERVES: 1**

LETTUCE SALAD

INGREDIENTS

- 1 cup Romaine lettuce, roughly chopped
- 3 oz seitan, chopped
- 1 tablespoon avocado oil
- 1 teaspoon sunflower seeds
- 1 teaspoon lemon juice
- 1 egg, boiled, peeled
- 2 oz Cheddar cheese, shredded

DIRECTIONS

1. Place lettuce in the salad bowl. Add chopped seitan and shredded cheese.
2. Then chop the egg roughly and add it in the salad bowl too.
3. Mix up together lemon juice with the avocado oil.
4. Sprinkle the salad with the oil mixture and sunflower seeds. Don't stir the salad before serving.

Nutritions: *Calories 20 Total Fat 0.2g Cholesterol 0mg Sodium 31mg Potassium 241mg Total Carbohydrates 4.2g Protein 1.2g*

PREPARATION: 10 MIN **COOKING: 25 MIN** **SERVES: 6**

ONION SOUP

INGREDIENTS

- 2 cups white onion, diced
- 4 tablespoon butter
- ½ cup white mushrooms, chopped
- 3 cups of water
- 1 cup heavy cream
- 1 teaspoon salt
- 1 teaspoon chili flakes
- 1 teaspoon garlic powder

DIRECTIONS

1. Put butter in the saucepan and melt it.
2. Add diced white onion, chili flakes, and garlic powder. Mix it up and saute for 10 minutes over medium-low heat.
3. Then add water, heavy cream, and chopped mushrooms. Close the lid.
4. Cook the soup for 15 minutes more.
5. Then blend the soup until you get the creamy texture. Ladle it in the bowls.

Nutritions: *Calories: 290. Fat: 9.6g. Protein: 16.8g. Carbohydrate: 33.4g.*

PREPARATION: 10 MIN **COOKING: 15 MIN** **SERVES: 3**

ASPARAGUS SALAD

INGREDIENTS

- 10 oz asparagus
- 1 tablespoon olive oil
- ½ teaspoon white pepper
- 4 oz Feta cheese, crumbled
- 1 cup lettuce, chopped
- 1 tablespoon canola oil
- 1 teaspoon apple cider vinegar
- 1 tomato, diced

DIRECTIONS

1. Preheat the oven to 365F.
2. Place asparagus in the tray, sprinkle with olive oil and white pepper, and transfer to the preheated oven. Cook it for 15 minutes.
3. Meanwhile, put crumbled Feta in the salad bowl.
4. Add chopped lettuce and diced tomato.
5. Sprinkle the ingredients with apple cider vinegar.
6. Chill the cooked asparagus to room temperature and add in the salad.
7. Shake the salad gently before serving.

Nutritions: *Calories: 87.5 Total Fat: 4.1 g Cholesterol: 9.2 mg Sodium: 685.8 mg Potassium: 212.1 mg Total Carbohydrate: 8.1 g Protein: 5.1 g*

PREPARATION: 5 MIN **COOKING: 18 MIN** **SERVES: 2**

BEEF WITH CABBAGE NOODLES

INGREDIENTS

- 4 oz ground beef
- 1 cup chopped cabbage
- 4 oz tomato sauce
- ½ tsp. minced garlic
- ½ cup of water

Seasoning:
- ½ tbsp.. coconut oil
- ½ tsp. salt
- ¼ tsp. Italian seasoning
- 1/8 tsp. dried basil

DIRECTIONS

1. Take a skillet pan, place it over medium heat, add oil and when hot, add beef and cook for 5 minutes until nicely browned.
2. Meanwhile, prepare the cabbage and, for it, slice the cabbage into thin shred.
3. When the beef has cooked, add garlic, season with salt, basil, and Italian seasoning, stir well and continue cooking for 3 minutes until the beef has thoroughly cooked.
4. Pour in tomato sauce and water, stir well and bring the mixture to boil.
5. Then reduce heat to medium-low level, add cabbage, stir well until well mixed and simmer for 3 to 5 minutes until cabbage is softened, covering the pan.
6. Uncover the pan and continue simmering the beef until most of the cooking liquid has evaporated.
7. Serve.

Nutritions: *Calories: 188.5 Fats: 12.5 g Protein: 15.5 g Net Carbohydrates: 2.5 g Fiber: 1 g*

PREPARATION: 5 MIN   **COOKING: 0 MIN**   **SERVES: 2**

ROAST BEEF AND MOZZARELLA PLATE

INGREDIENTS

- 4 slices of roast beef
- ½ ounce chopped lettuce
- 1 avocado, pitted
- 2 oz mozzarella cheese, cubed
- ½ cup mayonnaise

Seasoning:

- ¼ tsp. salt
- 1/8 tsp. ground black pepper
- 2 tbsp. avocado oil

DIRECTIONS

1. Scoop out flesh from avocado and divide it evenly between two plates.
2. Add slices of roast beef, lettuce, and cheese, and then sprinkle with salt and black pepper.
3. Serve with avocado oil and mayonnaise.

Nutritions: *Calories: 267.7 Fats: 24.5 g Protein: 9.5 g Net Carbohydrates: 1.5 g Fiber: 2 g*

| PREPARATION: 5 MIN | COOKING: 10 MIN | SERVES: 2 |

GARLIC HERB BEEF ROAST

INGREDIENTS

- 6 slices of beef roast
- ½ tsp. garlic powder
- 1/3 tsp. dried thyme
- ¼ tsp. dried rosemary
- 2 tbsp. butter, unsalted

Seasoning:
- 1/3 tsp. salt
- 1/4 tsp. ground black pepper

DIRECTIONS

1. Prepare the spice mix and for this, take a small bowl, place garlic powder, thyme, rosemary, salt, and black pepper and then stir until mixed.
2. Sprinkle spice mix on the beef roast.
3. Take a medium skillet pan, place it over medium heat, add butter and when it melts, add beef roast and then cook for 5 to 8 minutes until golden brown and cooked.
4. Serve.

Nutritions: *Calories: 140 Fats: 12.7 g Protein: 5.5 g Net Carbohydrates: 0.1 g Fiber: 0.2 g*

PREPARATION: 5 MIN **COOKING: 8 MIN** **SERVES: 2**

SPROUTS STIR-FRY WITH KALE, BROCCOLI, AND BEEF

INGREDIENTS

- 3 slices of beef roast, chopped
- 2 oz Brussels sprouts, halved
- 4 oz broccoli florets
- 3 oz kale
- 1 ½ tbsp.. butter, unsalted
- 1/8 tsp. red pepper flakes

Seasoning:
- ¼ tsp. garlic powder
- ¼ tsp. salt
- 1/8 tsp. ground black pepper

DIRECTIONS

1. Take a medium skillet pan, place it over medium heat, add ¾ tbsp. butter and when it melts, add broccoli florets and sprouts, sprinkle with garlic powder, and cook for 2 minutes.
2. Season vegetables with salt and red pepper flakes, add chopped beef, stir until mixed and continue cooking for 3 minutes until browned on one side.
3. Then add kale along with remaining butter, flip the vegetables and cook for 2 minutes until kale leaves wilts.
4. Serve.

Nutritions: *Calories: 125 Fats: 9.4 g Protein: 4.8 g Net Carbohydrates: 1.7 g Fiber: 2.6 g*

PREPARATION: 5 MIN **COOKING: 15 MIN** **SERVES: 2**

BEEF AND VEGETABLE SKILLET

INGREDIENTS

- 3 oz spinach, chopped
- ½ pound ground beef
- 2 slices of bacon, diced
- 2 oz chopped asparagus

Seasoning:
- 3 tbsp. coconut oil
- 2 tsp. dried thyme
- 2/3 tsp. salt
- ½ tsp. ground black pepper

DIRECTIONS

1. Take a skillet pan, place it over medium heat, add oil and when hot, add beef and bacon and cook for 5 to 7 minutes until slightly browned.
2. Then add asparagus and spinach, sprinkle with thyme, stir well and cook for 7 to 10 minutes until thoroughly cooked.
3. Season with salt and black pepper and serve.

Nutritions: *Calories 332.5 Fats 26 g; Protein 23.5 g; Carbohydrates 1.5 g Fiber 1 g*

PREPARATION: 5 MIN **COOKING: 18 MIN** **SERVES: 2**

BEEF, PEPPER AND GREEN BEANS STIR-FRY

INGREDIENTS

- 6 oz ground beef
- 2 oz chopped green bell pepper
- 4 oz green beans
- 3 tbsp. grated cheddar cheese

Seasoning:
- ½ tsp. salt
- ¼ tsp. ground black pepper
- ¼ tsp. paprika

DIRECTIONS

1. Take a skillet pan, place it over medium heat, add ground beef and cook for 4 minutes until slightly browned.
2. Then add bell pepper and green beans, season with salt, paprika, and black pepper, stir well and continue cooking for 7 to 10 minutes until beef and vegetables have cooked through.
3. Sprinkle cheddar cheese on top, then transfer pan under the broiler and cook for 2 minutes until cheese has melted and the top is golden brown.
4. Serve.

Nutritions: *Calories: 282.5 Fats: 17.6 g Protein: 26.1 g Net Carbohydrates: 2.9 g*

9. MEAT RECIPES

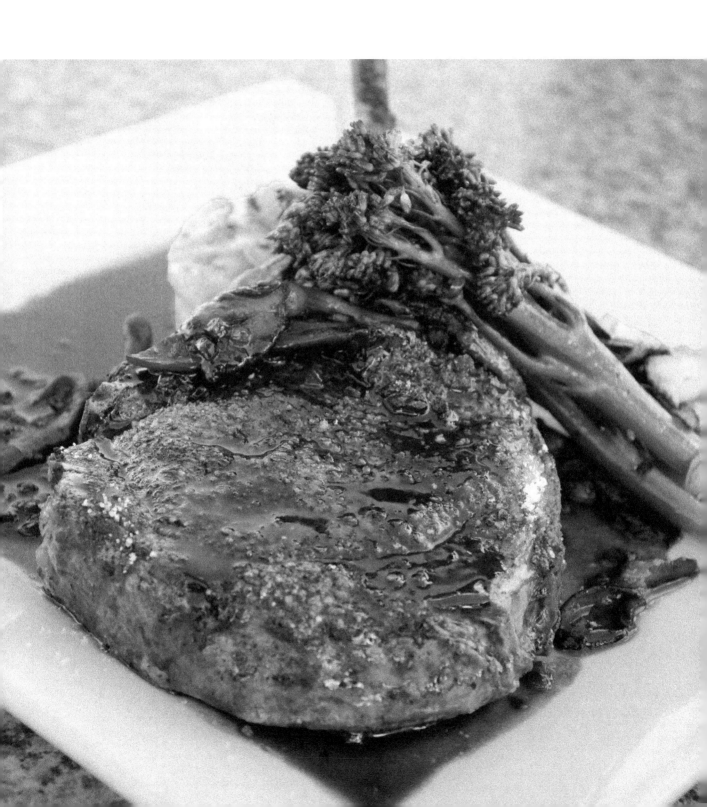

PREPARATION: 5 MIN **COOKING: 18 MIN** **SERVES: 2**

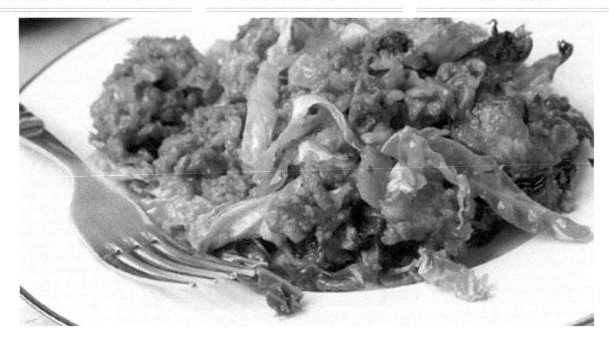

BEEF WITH CABBAGE NOODLES

INGREDIENTS

- 4 oz ground beef
- 1 cup chopped cabbage
- 4 oz tomato sauce
- ½ tsp. minced garlic
- ½ cup of water

Seasoning:
- ½ tbsp. coconut oil
- ½ tsp. salt
- ¼ tsp. Italian seasoning
- 1/8 tsp. dried basil

DIRECTIONS

1. Take a skillet pan, place it over medium heat, add oil and when hot, add beef and cook for 5 minutes until nicely browned.
2. Meanwhile, prepare the cabbage and for it slice the cabbage into thin shred.
3. When the beef has cooked, add garlic, season with salt, basil, and Italian seasoning, stir well and continue cooking for 3 minutes until the beef has thoroughly cooked.
4. Pour in tomato sauce and water, stir well and bring the mixture to boil.
5. Then reduce heat to medium-low level, add cabbage, stir well until well mixed and simmer for 3 to 5 minutes until cabbage is softened, covering the pan.
6. Uncover the pan and continue simmering the beef until most of the cooking liquid has evaporated.
7. Serve.

Nutritions: *188.5 Calories 12.5 g Fats 15.5 g Protein 2.5 g Net Carb 1 g Fiber*

PREPARATION: 5 MIN **COOKING: 0 MIN** **SERVES: 2**

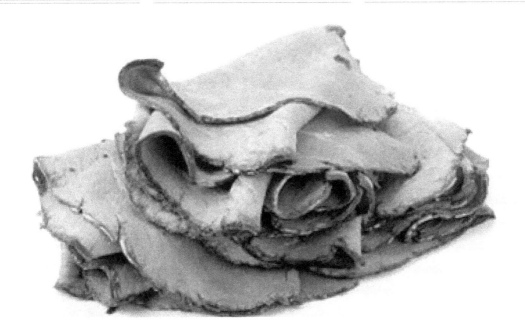

ROAST BEEF AND MOZZARELLA PLATE

INGREDIENTS

- 4 slices of roast beef
- ½ ounce chopped lettuce
- 1 avocado, pitted
- 2 oz mozzarella cheese, cubed
- ½ cup mayonnaise

Seasoning:
- ¼ tsp. salt
- 1/8 tsp. ground black pepper
- 2 tbsp. avocado oil

DIRECTIONS

1. Scoop out flesh from the avocado and divide it evenly between two plates.
2. Add slices of roast beef, lettuce, and cheese, and then sprinkle with salt and black pepper.
3. Serve with avocado oil and mayonnaise.

Nutritions: *267.7 Calories 24.5 g Fats 9.5 g Protein 1.5 g Net Carb 2 g Fiber*

PREPARATION: 5 MIN **COOKING: 10 MIN** **SERVES: 2**

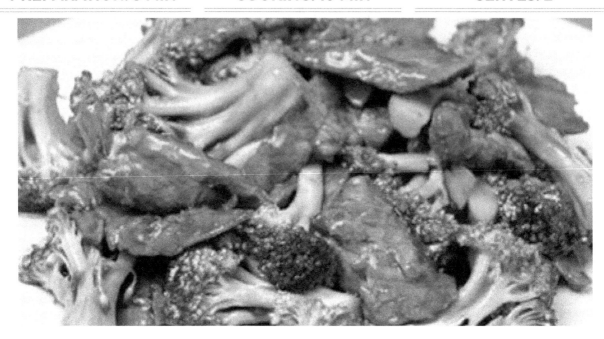

BEEF AND BROCCOLI

INGREDIENTS

- 6 slices of beef roast, cut into strips
- 1 scallion, chopped
- 3 oz broccoli florets, chopped
- 1 tbsp. avocado oil
- 1 tbsp. butter, unsalted

Seasoning:
- ¼ tsp. salt
- 1/8 tsp. ground black pepper
- 1 ½ tbsp. soy sauce
- 3 tbsp. chicken broth

DIRECTIONS

1. Take a medium skillet pan, place it over medium heat, add oil and when hot, add beef strips and cook for 2 minutes until hot.
2. Transfer beef to a plate, add scallion to the pan, then add butter and cook for 3 minutes until tender.
3. Add remaining ingredients, stir until mixed, switch heat to the low level, and simmer for 3 to 4 minutes until broccoli is tender.
4. Return beef to the pan, stir until well combined, and cook for 1 minute.
5. Serve.

Nutritions: *245 Calories 15.7 g Fats 21.6 g Protein 1.7 g Net Carb 1.3 g Fiber*

PREPARATION: 5 MIN   **COOKING: 10 MIN**   **SERVES: 2**

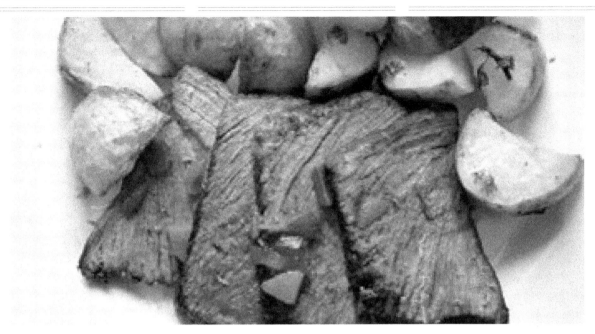

GARLIC HERB BEEF ROAST

INGREDIENTS

- 6 slices of beef roast
- ½ tsp. garlic powder
- 1/3 tsp. dried thyme
- ¼ tsp. dried rosemary
- 2 tbsp. butter, unsalted

Seasoning:
- 1/3 tsp. salt
- 1/4 tsp. ground black pepper

DIRECTIONS

1. Prepare the spice mix and for this, take a small bowl, place garlic powder, thyme, rosemary, salt, and black pepper and then stir until mixed.
2. Sprinkle spice mix on the beef roast.
3. Take a medium skillet pan, place it over medium heat, add butter and when it melts, add beef roast and then cook for 5 to 8 minutes until golden brown and cooked.
4. Serve.

Nutritions: *140 Calories 12.7 g Fats 5.5 g Protein 0.1 g Net Carb 0.2 g Fiber*

PREPARATION: 5 MIN **COOKING: 8 MIN** **SERVES: 2**

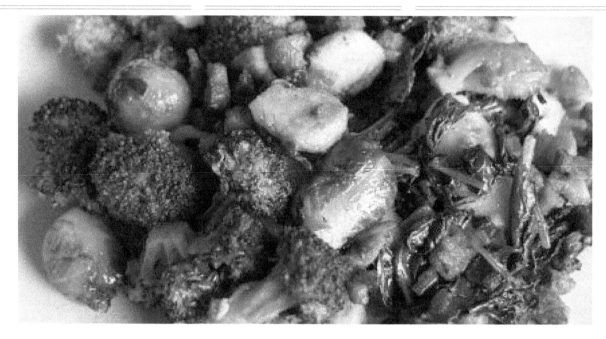

SPROUTS STIR-FRY WITH KALE, BROCCOLI, AND BEEF

INGREDIENTS

- 3 slices of beef roast, chopped
- 2 oz Brussels sprouts, halved
- 4 oz broccoli florets
- 3 oz kale
- 1 ½ tbsp. butter, unsalted
- 1/8 tsp. red pepper flakes

Seasoning:
- ¼ tsp. garlic powder
- ¼ tsp. salt
- 1/8 tsp. ground black pepper

DIRECTIONS

1. Take a medium skillet pan, place it over medium heat, add ¾ tbsp butter and when it melts, add broccoli florets and sprouts, sprinkle with garlic powder, and cook for 2 minutes.
2. Season vegetables with salt and red pepper flakes, add chopped beef, stir until mixed and continue cooking for 3 minutes until browned on one side.
3. Then add kale along with remaining butter, flip the vegetables and cook for 2 minutes until kale leaves wilt.
4. Serve.

Nutritions: *125 Calories 9.4 g Fats 4.8 g Protein 1.7 g Net Carb 2.6 g Fiber*

PREPARATION: 5 MIN **COOKING: 15 MIN** **SERVES: 2**

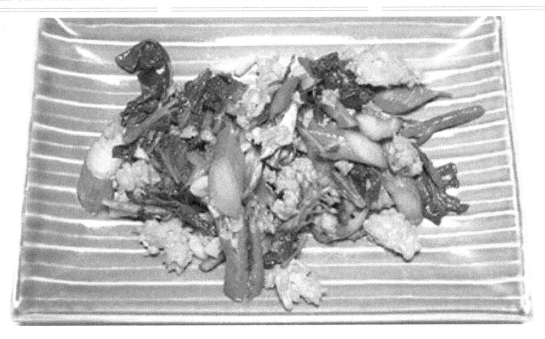

BEEF AND VEGETABLE SKILLET

INGREDIENTS

- 3 oz spinach, chopped
- ½ pound ground beef
- 2 slices of bacon, diced
- 2 oz chopped asparagus

Seasoning:
- 3 tbsp. coconut oil
- 2 tsp. dried thyme
- 2/3 tsp. salt
- ½ tsp. ground black pepper

DIRECTIONS

1. Take a skillet pan, place it over medium heat, add oil and when hot, add beef and bacon and cook for 5 to 7 minutes until slightly browned.
2. Then add asparagus and spinach, sprinkle with thyme, stir well and cook for 7 to 10 minutes until thoroughly cooked.
3. Season skillet with salt and black pepper and serve.

Nutritions: *332.5 Calories 26 g Fats 23.5 g Protein 1.5 g Net Carb 1 g Fiber*

PREPARATION: 5 MIN　　　**COOKING: 18 MIN**　　　**SERVES: 2**

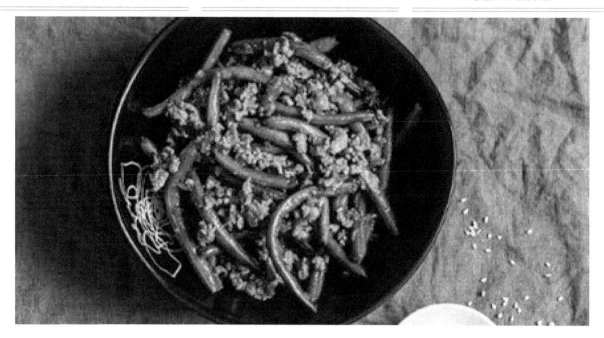

BEEF, PEPPER AND GREEN BEANS STIR-FRY

INGREDIENTS

- 6 oz ground beef
- 2 oz chopped green bell pepper
- 4 oz green beans
- 3 tbsp. grated cheddar cheese

Seasoning:
- ½ tsp. salt
- ¼ tsp. ground black pepper
- ¼ tsp. paprika

DIRECTIONS

1. Take a skillet pan, place it over medium heat, add ground beef and cook for 4 minutes until slightly browned.
2. Then add bell pepper and green beans, season with salt, paprika, and black pepper, stir well and continue cooking for 7 to 10 minutes until beef and vegetables have cooked through.
3. Sprinkle cheddar cheese on top, then transfer pan under the broiler and cook for 2 minutes until cheese has melted and the top is golden brown.
4. Serve.

Nutritions: *282.5 Calories 17.6 g Fats 26.1 g Protein 2.9 g Net Carb 2.1 g Fiber*

PREPARATION: 5 MIN **COOKING: 4 MIN** **SERVES: 2**

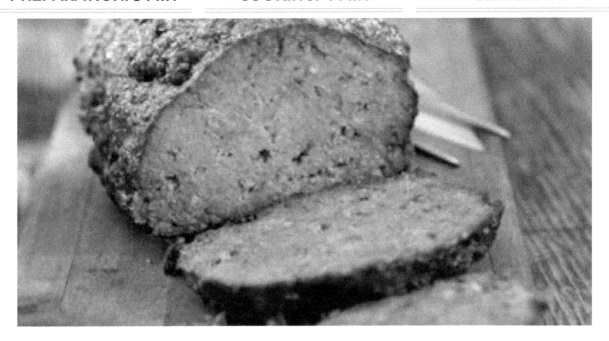

CHEESY MEATLOAF

INGREDIENTS

- 4 oz ground turkey
- 1 egg
- 1 tbsp. grated mozzarella cheese
- ¼ tsp. Italian seasoning
- ½ tbsp. soy sauce

Seasoning:
- ¼ tsp. salt
- 1/8 tsp. ground black pepper

DIRECTIONS

1. Take a bowl, place all the ingredients in it, and stir until mixed.
2. Take a heatproof mug, spoon in prepared mixture, and microwave for 3 minutes at high heat setting until cooked.
3. When done, let meatloaf rest in the mug for 1 minute, then take it out, cut it into two slices, and serve.

Nutritions: *196.5 Calories 13.5 g Fats 18.7 g Protein 18.7 g Net Carb 0 g Fiber*

PREPARATION: 10 MIN **COOKING: 10 MIN** **SERVES: 2**

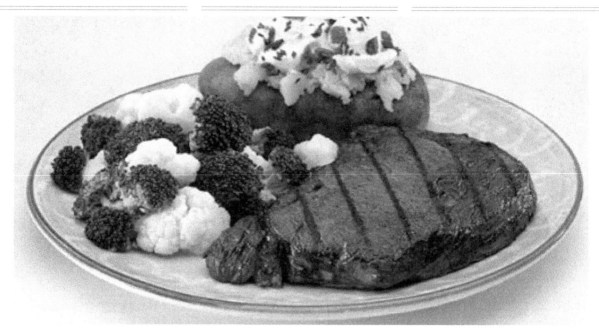

ROAST BEEF AND VEGETABLE PLATE

INGREDIENTS

- 2 scallions, chopped into large pieces
- 1 ½ tbsp. coconut oil
- 4 thin slices of roast beef
- 4 oz cauliflower and broccoli mix
- 1 tbsp. butter, unsalted

Seasoning:
- 1/2 tsp. salt
- 1/3 tsp. ground black pepper
- 1 tsp. dried parsley

DIRECTIONS

1. Turn on the oven, then set it to 400 degrees F, and let it preheat.
2. Take a baking sheet, grease it with oil, place slices of roast beef on one side, and top with butter.
3. Take a separate bowl, add cauliflower and broccoli mix, add scallions, drizzle with oil, season with remaining salt and black pepper, toss until coated, and then spread vegetables on the empty side of the baking sheet.
4. Bake for 5 to 7 minutes until beef is nicely browned and vegetables are tender-crisp, tossing halfway.
5. Distribute beef and vegetables between two plates and then serve.

Nutritions: *313 Calories 26 g Fats 15.6 g Protein 2.8 g Net Carb 1.9 g Fiber*

PREPARATION: 5 MIN   **COOKING: 10 MIN**   **SERVES: 2**

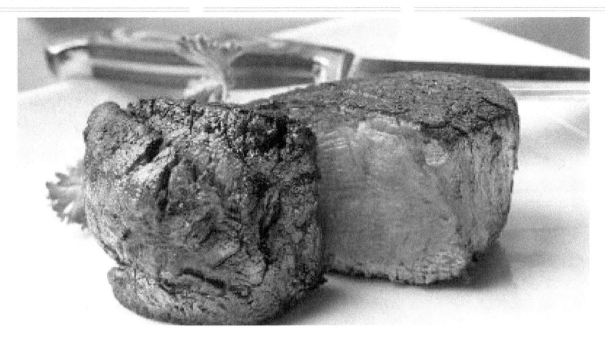

STEAK AND CHEESE PLATE

INGREDIENTS

- 1 green onion, chopped
- 2 oz chopped lettuce
- 2 beef steaks
- 2 oz of cheddar cheese, sliced
- ½ cup mayonnaise

Seasoning:
- ¼ tsp salt
- 1/8 tsp ground black pepper
- 3 tbsp avocado oil

DIRECTIONS

1. Prepare the steak, and for this, season it with salt and black pepper.
2. Take a medium skillet pan, place it over medium heat, add oil, and when hot, add seasoned steaks and cook for 7 to 10 minutes until cooked to the desired level.
3. When done, distribute steaks between two plates, add scallion, lettuce, and cheese slices.
4. Drizzle with remaining oil and then serve with mayonnaise.

Nutritions: *714 Calories 65.3 g Fats 25.3 g Protein 4 g Net Carb 5.3 g Fiber*

PREPARATION: 15 MIN   **COOKING: 12 MIN**   **SERVES: 2**

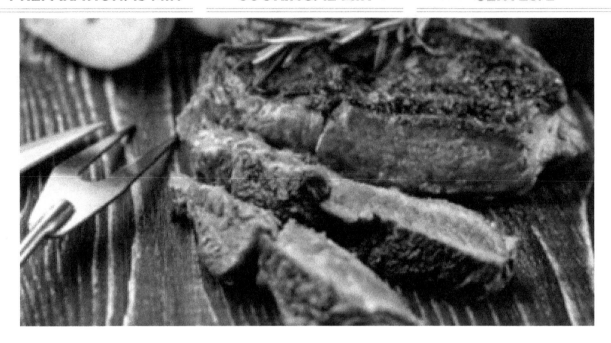

GARLICKY STEAKS WITH ROSEMARY

INGREDIENTS

- 2 beef steaks
- 1/4 of a lime, juiced
- 1 ½ tsp. garlic powder
- ¾ tsp. dried rosemary
- 2 ½ tbsp. avocado oil

Seasoning:
- ½ tsp. salt
- ¼ tsp. ground black pepper

DIRECTIONS

1. Prepare steaks, and for this, sprinkle garlic powder on all sides of the steak.
2. Take a shallow dish, place 1 ½ tbsp oil and lime juice in it, whisk until combined, add steaks, turn to coat and let it marinate for 20 minutes at room temperature.
3. Then take a griddle pan, place it over medium-high heat and grease it with remaining oil.
4. Season marinated steaks with salt and black pepper, add to the griddle pan, and cook for 7 to 12 minutes until cooked to the desired level.
5. When done, wrap steaks in foil for 5 minutes, then cut into slices across the grain.
6. Sprinkle rosemary over steaks slices and then serve.

Nutritions: *213 Calories 13 g Fats 22 g Protein 1 g Net Carb 0 g Fiber*

10. FISH SEAFOOD

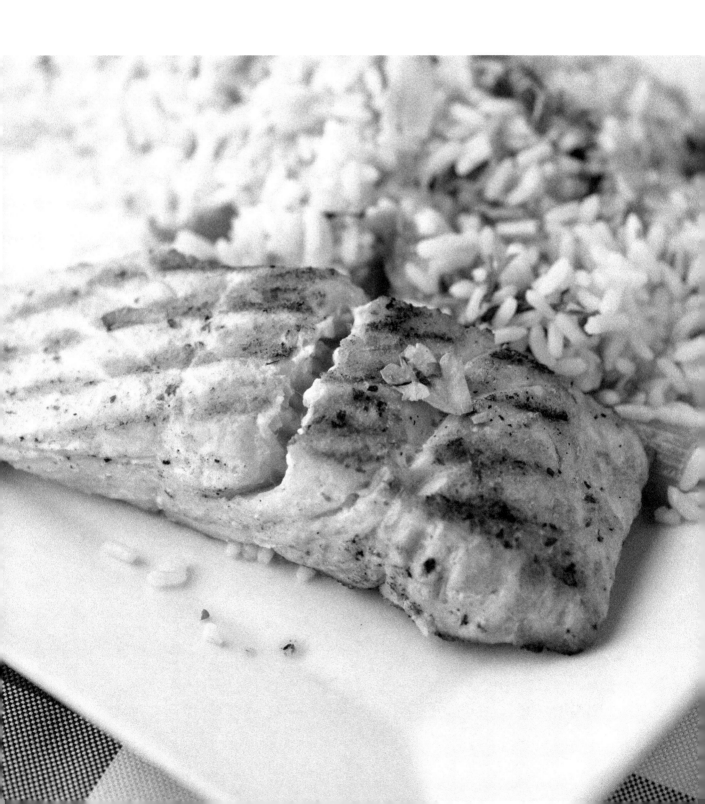

PREPARATION: 15 MIN **COOKING: 10 MIN** **SERVES: 4**

SWEET & SOUR GROUPER

INGREDIENTS

- 2 tbsp. Scallion, chopped
- ¾ tsp. fresh ginger root, minced
- 1-2 tbsp. garlic, minced
- ¼ C. olive oil
- 2 tbsp. balsamic vinegar
- 2 tbsp. low-sodium soy sauce
- 1 tsp. Powdered Erythritol
- ½ tsp. red pepper flakes, crushed
- Salt, to taste
- 4 (6-oz.) grouper fillets

DIRECTIONS

1. Mix all fixing except grouper fillets in a large bowl.
2. Add the grouper fillets and coat with the marinade generously.
3. Chill, and marinate for about 8 hours, tossing occasionally.
4. Preheat the grill to medium-high heat. Grease the grill grate.
5. Place the grouper fillets onto the grill about 5-inch away from the heat source.
6. Cook for about 7-10 minutes, flipping once or until the desired doneness halfway through.
7. Serve hot.

Nutritions: *Calories: 318 Carbohydrates: 1.7g Protein: 43g Fat: 14.9g*

| PREPARATION: 10 MIN | COOKING: 13 MIN | SERVES: 2 |

AROMATIC COD

INGREDIENTS

- 2 (6-oz.) cod fillets
- 1 tsp. onion powder
- Salt
- Ground black pepper
- 3 tbsp. butter, divided
- 2 garlic cloves, minced
- 1-2 lemon slices
- 2 tsp. fresh dill weed

DIRECTIONS

1. Season each cod fillet evenly with the onion powder, salt, and black pepper.
2. Dissolve 1 tbsp. of butter over high heat and cook the cod fillets for about 4-5 minutes per side.
3. Transfer the cod fillets onto a plate.
4. Meanwhile, in a frying pan, melt the remaining butter over low heat and sauté the garlic and lemon slices for about 40-60 seconds.
5. Stir in the cooked cod fillets and dill and cook, covered for about 1-2 minutes.
6. Remove the cod fillets from heat and transfer onto the serving plates.
7. Top with the pan sauce and serve immediately.

Nutritions: *Calories: 301 Carbohydrates: 2.5g Protein: 31.1g Fat: 18.9g*

PREPARATION: 15 MIN **COOKING: 20 MIN** **SERVES: 4**

FLAVORSOME COD BAKE

INGREDIENTS

- 1 tsp. olive oil
- ½ C. yellow onion, minced
- 1 C. zucchini, chopped
- 1 garlic clove, minced
- 2 tbsp. fresh basil, chopped
- 2 C. fresh tomatoes
- Salt
- Ground black pepper
- 4 (6-oz.) cod steaks
- 1/3 C. feta cheese, crumbled

DIRECTIONS

1. Heat-up the oven to 450 degrees F, then grease a large shallow baking dish.
2. In a skillet, heat the oil over medium heat and sauté the onion, zucchini, and garlic for about 4-5 minutes.
3. Stir in the basil, tomatoes, salt, and black pepper, and immediately remove from the heat.
4. Place the cod steaks into a prepared baking dish in a single layer and top with the tomato mixture.
5. Sprinkle with the feta cheese evenly. Bake for 15 minutes, remove the cod mixture from the oven, and serve hot.

Nutritions: *Calories: 250 Carbohydrates: 6.6g Protein: 42g Fat: 5.5g*

| PREPARATION: 15 MIN | COOKING: 25 MIN | SERVES: 6 |

SUPER-SIMPLE TROUT

INGREDIENTS

- 2 (1½-lb.) wild-caught trout, gutted and cleaned
- Salt
- Ground black pepper
- 1 lemon, sliced
- 2 tbsp. fresh dill, minced
- 2 tbsp. butter, melted
- 2 tbsp. lemon juice

DIRECTIONS

1. Heat-up the oven to 475 degrees F. Put the trout plus salt and pepper.
2. Load the fish cavity with lemon slices and dill. Drizzle the trout with the melted butter and lemon juice.
3. Bake for about 25 minutes.
4. Serve hot.

Nutritions: *Calories: 469 Carbohydrates: 0.9g Protein: 60.7g Fat: 23.1g*

11. SNACKS

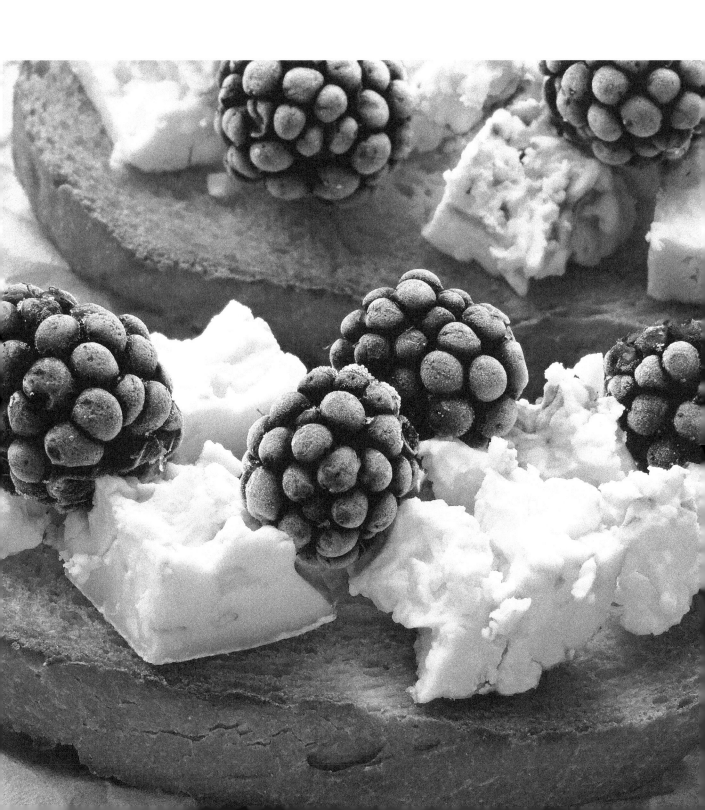

PREPARATION: 20 MIN **COOKING: 60 MIN** **SERVES: 12**

KORMA CURRY

INGREDIENTS

- 2 teaspoons cinnamon
- 2/3 cup sour cream
- 2 cups heavy cream
- 1 teaspoon scraped vanilla bean
- ¼ teaspoon cardamom
- 4 egg yolks
- Stevia to taste

DIRECTIONS

1. Start by whisking your egg yolks until creamy and smooth.
2. Get out a double boiler, and add your eggs with the rest of your ingredients. Mix well.
3. Remove from heat, allowing it to cool until it reaches room temperature.
4. Refrigerate for an hour before whisking well.
5. Pour into molds, and freeze for at least an hour before serving.

Nutritions: *Calories: 363 Protein: 2 Fat: 40 Carbohydrates: 1*

PREPARATION: 20 MIN **COOKING: 60 MIN** **SERVES: 12**

COCONUT FUDGE

INGREDIENTS

- 2 cups coconut oil
- ½ cup dark cocoa powder
- ½ cup coconut cream
- ¼ cup almonds, chopped
- ¼ cup coconut, shredded
- 1 teaspoon almond extract
- Pinch of salt
- Stevia to taste

DIRECTIONS

1. Pour your coconut oil and coconut cream into a bowl, whisking with an electric beater until smooth. Once the mixture becomes smooth and glossy, do not continue.
2. Begin to add in your cocoa powder while mixing slowly, making sure that there aren't any lumps.
3. Add in the rest of your ingredients, and mix well.
4. Line a bread pan with parchment paper, and freeze until it sets.
5. Slice into squares before serving.

Nutritions: *Calories: 172 Fat: 20 Carbohydrates: 3*

PREPARATION: 30 MIN **COOKING: 60 MIN** **SERVES: 12**

NUTMEG NOUGAT

INGREDIENTS

- 1 cup heavy cream
- 1 cup cashew butter
- 1 cup coconut, shredded
- ½ teaspoon nutmeg
- 1 teaspoon vanilla extract, pure
- Stevia to taste

DIRECTIONS

1. Melt your cashew butter using a double boiler, and then stir in your vanilla extract, dairy cream, nutmeg, and stevia. Make sure it's mixed well.
2. Remove from heat, allowing it to cool down before refrigerating it for a half-hour.
3. Shape into balls, and coat with shredded coconut. Chill for at least two hours before serving.

Nutritions: *Calories: 341 Fat: 34 Carbohydrates: 5*

| PREPARATION: 30 MIN | COOKING: 90 MIN | SERVES: 12 |

SWEET ALMOND BITES

INGREDIENTS

- 18 ounces butter, grass-fed
- 2 ounces heavy cream
- ½ cup Stevia
- 2/3 cup cocoa powder
- 1 teaspoon vanilla extract, pure
- 4 tablespoons almond butter

DIRECTIONS

1. Use a double boiler to melt your butter before adding in all of your remaining ingredients.
2. Place the mixture into molds, freezing for two hours before serving.

Nutritions: *Calories: 350 Protein: 2 Fat: 38*

| PREPARATION: 30 MIN | COOKING: 12 | SERVES: 12 |

STRAWBERRY CHEESECAKE MINIS

INGREDIENTS

- 1 cup coconut oil
- 1 cup coconut butter
- ½ cup strawberries, sliced
- ½ teaspoon lime juice
- 2 tablespoons cream cheese, full fat
- Stevia to taste

DIRECTIONS

1. Blend your strawberries together.
2. Soften your cream cheese, and then add in your coconut butter.
3. Combine all ingredients together, and then pour your mixture into silicone molds.
4. Freeze for at least two hours before serving.

Nutritions: *Calories: 372 Protein: 1 Fat: 41 Carbohydrates: 2*

PREPARATION: 10 MIN **COOKING: 30 MIN** **SERVES: 12**

COCOA BROWNIES

INGREDIENTS

- 1 egg
- 2 tablespoons butter, grass-fed
- 2 teaspoons vanilla extract, pure
- ¼ teaspoon baking powder
- ¼ cup cocoa powder
- 1/3 cup heavy cream
- ¾ cup almond butter
- Pinch sea salt

DIRECTIONS

1. Break your egg into a bowl, whisking until smooth.
2. Add in all of your wet ingredients, mixing well.
3. Mix all dry ingredients into a bowl.
4. Sift your dry ingredients into your wet ingredients, mixing to form a batter.
5. Get out a baking pan, greasing it before pouring in your mixture.
6. Heat your oven to 350 and bake for twenty-five minutes.
7. Allow it to cool before slicing and serve room temperature or warm.

Nutritions: *Calories: 184 Protein: 1 Fat: 20 Carbohydrates: 1*

PREPARATION: 20 MIN **COOKING: 120 MIN** **SERVES: 6**

CHOCOLATE ORANGE BITES

INGREDIENTS

- 10 ounces coconut oil
- 4 tablespoons cocoa powder
- ¼ teaspoon blood orange extract
- Stevia to taste

DIRECTIONS

1. Melt half of your coconut oil using a double boiler, and then add in your stevia and orange extract.
2. Get out candy molds, pouring the mixture into it. Fill each mold halfway, and then place in the fridge until they set.
3. Melt the other half of your coconut oil, stirring in your cocoa powder and stevia, making sure that the mixture is smooth with no lumps.
4. Pour into your molds, filling them up all the way, and then allow it to set in the fridge before serving.

Nutritions: *Calories: 188 Protein: 1 Fat: 21 Carbohydrates: 5*

PREPARATION: 25 MIN **COOKING: 120 MIN** **SERVES: 6**

CARAMEL CONES

INGREDIENTS

- 2 tablespoons heavy whipping cream
- 2 tablespoons sour cream
- 1 tablespoon caramel sugar
- 1 teaspoon sea salt, fine
- 1/3 cup butter, grass-fed
- 1/3 cup coconut oil
- Stevia to taste

DIRECTIONS

1. Soften your coconut oil and butter, mixing.
2. Mix all ingredients to form a batter, and then place them in molds.
3. Top with a little salt, and keep refrigerated until serving.

Nutritions: *Calories: 100 Fat: 12 Grams Carbohydrates: 1*

PREPARATION: 20 MIN **COOKING: 95 MIN** **SERVES: 6**

CINNAMON BITES

INGREDIENTS

- 1/8 teaspoon nutmeg
- 1 teaspoon vanilla extract
- ¼ teaspoon cinnamon
- 4 tablespoons coconut oil
- ½ cup butter, grass-fed
- 8 ounces cream cheese
- Stevia to taste

DIRECTIONS

1. Soften your coconut oil and butter, mixing in your cream cheese.
2. Add all of your remaining ingredients, and mix well.
3. Pour into molds, and freeze until set.

Nutritions: *Calories: 178 Protein: 1 Fat: 19*

PREPARATION: 20 MIN **COOKING: 45 MIN** **SERVES: 6**

SWEET CHAI BITES

INGREDIENTS

- 1 cup cream cheese
- 1 cup coconut oil
- 2 ounces butter, grass-fed
- 2 teaspoons ginger
- 2 teaspoons cardamom
- 1 teaspoon nutmeg
- 1 teaspoon cloves
- 1 teaspoon vanilla extract, pure
- 1 teaspoon darjeeling black tea
- Stevia to taste

DIRECTIONS

1. Melt your coconut oil and butter before adding in your black tea. Allow it to set for one to two minutes.
2. Add in your cream cheese, removing your mixture from heat.
3. Add in all of your spices, and stir to combine.
4. Pour into molds, and freeze before serving.

Nutritions: *Calories: 178 Protein: 1 Fat: 19*

| PREPARATION: 20 MIN | COOKING: 45 MIN | SERVES: 14 |

EASY VANILLA BOMBS

INGREDIENTS

- 1 cup macadamia nuts, unsalted
- ¼ cup coconut oil / ¼ cup butter
- 2 teaspoons vanilla extract, sugar-free
- 20 drops liquid Stevia
- 2 tablespoons erythritol, powdered

DIRECTIONS

1. Pulse your macadamia nuts in a blender, and then combine all of your ingredients together. Mix well.
2. Get out mini muffin tins with a tablespoon and a half of the mixture.
3. Refrigerate it for a half-hour before serving.

Nutritions: *Calories:125 Fat: 5 Carbohydrates: 5*

PREPARATION: 2H 10 MIN **COOKING: 7 MIN** **SERVES: 4**

MARINATED EGGS

INGREDIENTS

- 6 eggs
- 1 and ¼ cups of water
- ¼ cup unsweetened rice vinegar
- 2 tablespoons coconut aminos
- Salt and black pepper to the taste
- 2 garlic cloves, minced
- 1 teaspoon stevia
- 4 ounces cream cheese
- 1 tablespoon chives, chopped

DIRECTIONS

1. Put the eggs in a pot, add water to cover, bring to a boil over medium heat, cover and cook for 7 minutes.
2. Rinse eggs with cold water and leave them aside to cool down.
3. In a bowl, mix 1 cup water with coconut aminos, vinegar, stevia, and garlic and whisk well.
4. Put the eggs in this mix, cover with a kitchen towel, and leave them aside for 2 hours, rotating from time to time.
5. Peel eggs, cut in halves, and put egg yolks in a bowl.
6. Add ¼ cup water, cream cheese, salt, pepper, and chives and stir well.
7. Stuff egg whites with this mix and serve them.
8. Enjoy!

Nutritions: *Calories: 289 kcal Protein: 15.86 g Fat: 22.62 g Carbohydrates: 4.52 g Sodium: 288 mg*

PREPARATION: 10 MIN **COOKING: 130 MIN** **SERVES: 28**

SAUSAGE AND CHEESE DIP

INGREDIENTS

- 8 ounces cream cheese
- A pinch of salt and black pepper
- 16 ounces sour cream
- 8 ounces pepper jack cheese, chopped
- 15 ounces canned tomatoes mixed with habaneros
- 1 pound Italian sausage, ground
- ¼ cup green onions, chopped

DIRECTIONS

1. Heat up a pan over medium heat, add sausage, stir and cook until it browns.
2. Add tomatoes mix, stir and cook for 4 minutes more.
3. Add a pinch of salt, pepper, and green onions, stir and cook for 4 minutes.
4. Spread pepper jack cheese on the bottom of your slow cooker.
5. Add cream cheese, sausage mix, and sour cream, cover, and cook on high for 2 hours.
6. Uncover your slow cooker, stir dip, transfer to a bowl, and serve.
7. Enjoy!

Nutritions: *Calories: 132 kcal Protein: 6.79 g Fat: 9.58 g Carbohydrates: 6.22 g Sodium: 362 mg*

PREPARATION: 20 MIN **COOKING: 30 MIN** **SERVES: 24**

TASTY ONION AND CAULIFLOWER DIP

INGREDIENTS

- 1 and ½ cups chicken stock
- 1 cauliflower head, florets separated
- ¼ cup mayonnaise
- ½ cup yellow onion, chopped
- ¾ cup cream cheese
- ½ teaspoon chili powder
- ½ teaspoon cumin, ground
- ½ teaspoon garlic powder
- Salt and black pepper to the taste

DIRECTIONS

1. Put the stock in a pot, add cauliflower and onion, heat up over medium heat and, cook for 30 minutes.
2. Add chili powder, salt, pepper, cumin, and garlic powder and stir.
3. Also, add cream cheese and stir a bit until it melts.
4. Blend using an immersion blender and mix with the mayo.
5. Transfer to a bowl and keep in the fridge for 2 hours before you serve it.
6. Enjoy!

Nutritions: *Calories: 40 kcal Protein: 1.23 g Fat: 3.31 g Carbohydrates: 1.66 g Sodium: 72 mg*

PREPARATION: 10 MIN **COOKING: 17 MIN** **SERVES: 6**

PESTO CRACKERS

INGREDIENTS

- ½ teaspoon baking powder
- Salt and black pepper to the taste
- 1 and ¼ cups almond flour
- ¼ teaspoon basil, dried
- 1 garlic clove, minced
- 2 tablespoons basil pesto
- A pinch of cayenne pepper
- 3 tablespoons ghee

DIRECTIONS

1. In a bowl, mix salt, pepper, baking powder, and almond flour.
2. Add garlic, cayenne, and basil and stir.
3. Add pesto and whisk.
4. Also, add ghee and mix your dough with your finger.
5. Spread this dough on a lined baking sheet, introduce in the oven at 325 degrees F and bake for 17 minutes.
6. Leave aside to cool down, cut your crackers, and serve them as a snack.
7. Enjoy!

Nutritions: Calories: 9 kcal Protein: 0.41 g Fat: 0.14 g Carbohydrates: 1.86 g Sodium: 2 mg

PREPARATION: 10 MIN **COOKING: 15 MIN** **SERVES: 18**

PUMPKIN MUFFINS

INGREDIENTS

- ¼ cup sunflower seed butter
- ¾ cup pumpkin puree
- 2 tablespoons flaxseed meal
- ¼ cup coconut flour
- ½ cup erythritol
- ½ teaspoon nutmeg, grounded
- 1 teaspoon cinnamon, grounded
- ½ teaspoon baking soda
- 1 egg
- ½ teaspoon baking powder
- A pinch of salt

DIRECTIONS

1. In a bowl, mix butter with pumpkin puree and egg and blend well.
2. Add flaxseed meal, coconut flour, erythritol, baking soda, baking powder, nutmeg, cinnamon, and a pinch of salt and stir well.
3. Spoon this into a greased muffin pan, introduce in the oven at 350 degrees F and bake for 15 minutes.
4. Leave muffins to cool down and serve them as a snack.
5. Enjoy!

Nutritions: *Calories: 65 kcal Protein: 2.82 g Fat: 5.42 g Carbohydrates: 2.27 g Sodium: 57 mg*

12. DESSERT

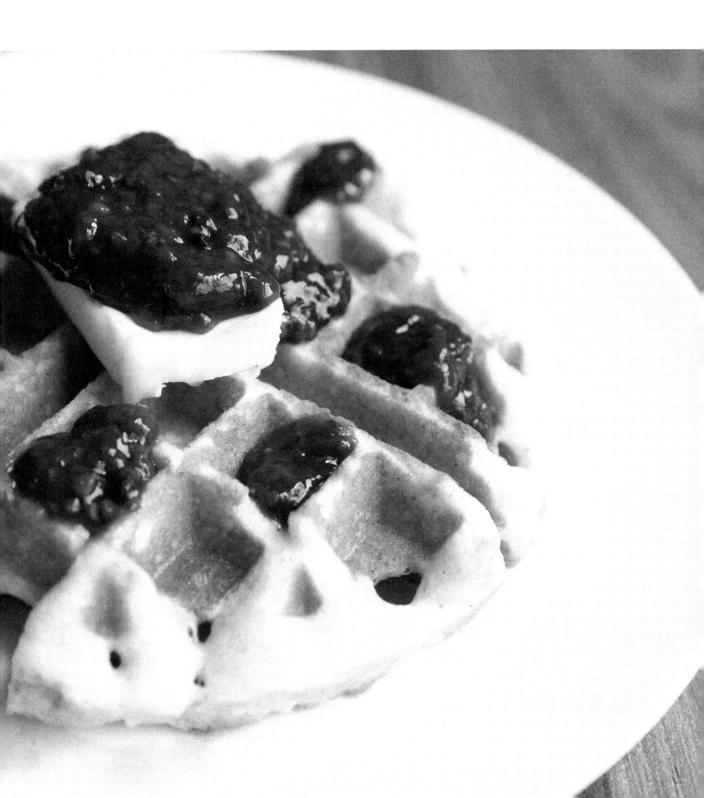

PREPARATION: 15 MIN **COOKING: 45 MIN** **SERVES: 8**

SUGAR-FREE LEMON BARS

INGREDIENTS

- ½ cup butter, melted
- 1¾ cup almond flour, divided
- 1 cup powdered erythritol, divided
- 3 medium-size lemons
- 3 large eggs

DIRECTIONS

1. Prepare the parchment paper and baking tray. Combine butter, 1 cup of almond flour, ¼ cup of erythritol, and salt. Stir well. Place the mix on the baking sheet, press a little, and put it into the oven (preheated to 350°F). Cook for about 20 minutes. Then set aside to let it cool.
2. Zest 1 lemon and juice all of the lemons in a bowl. Add the eggs, ¾ cup of erythritol, ¾ cup of almond flour, and salt. Stir together to create the filling. Pour it on top of the cake and cook for 25 minutes. Cut into small pieces and serve with lemon slices.

Nutritions: *Carbohydrates – 4 g Fat – 26 g Protein – 8 g Calories – 272*

PREPARATION: 5 MIN   **COOKING: 5 MIN**   **SERVES: 4**

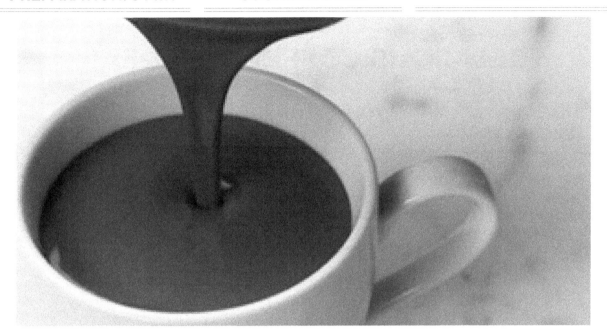

CREAMY HOT CHOCOLATE

INGREDIENTS

- 6 oz. dark chocolate, chopped
- ½ cup unsweetened almond milk
- ½ cup heavy cream
- 1 Tbsp. Erythritol
- ½ tsp. vanilla extract

DIRECTIONS

1. Combine the almond milk, erythritol, and cream in a small saucepan. Heat it (choose medium heat and cook for 1-2 minutes).
2. Add vanilla extract and chocolate. Stir continuously until the chocolate melts.
3. Pour into cups and serve.

Nutritions: *Carbohydrates – 4 g Fat – 18 g Protein – 2 g Calories – 193*

PREPARATION: 10 MIN **COOKING: 5 MIN** **SERVES: 1**

DELICIOUS COFFEE ICE CREAM

INGREDIENTS

- 6 ounces coconut cream, frozen into ice cubes
- 1 ripe avocado, diced and frozen
- ½ cup coffee expresso
- 2 Tbsp. sweetener
- 1 tsp. vanilla extract
- 1 Tbsp. water
- Coffee beans

DIRECTIONS

1. Take out the frozen coconut cubes and avocado from the fridge. Slightly melt them for 5-10 minutes.
2. Add the sweetener, coffee expresso, and vanilla extract to the coconut-avocado mix and whisk with an immersion blender until it becomes creamy (for about 1 minute). Pour in the water and blend for 30 seconds.
3. Top with coffee beans and enjoy!

Nutritions: *Carbohydrates – 20.5 g Fat – 61 g Protein – 6.3 g Calories – 596*

PREPARATION: 10 MIN **COOKING: 35 MIN** **SERVES: 10**

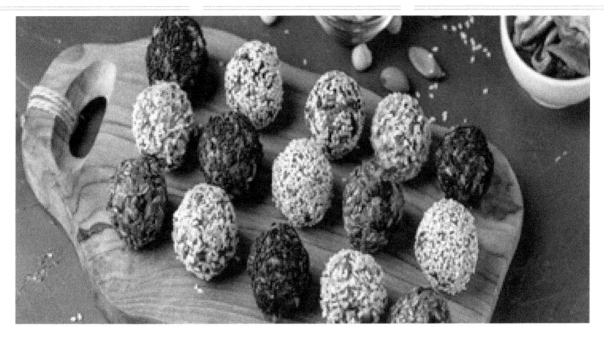

FATTY BOMBS WITH CINNAMON AND CARDAMOM

INGREDIENTS

- ½ cup unsweetened coconut, shredded
- 3 oz unsalted butter
- ¼ tsp. ground green cinnamon
- ¼ ground cardamom
- ½ tsp. vanilla extract

DIRECTIONS

1. Roast the unsweetened coconut (choose medium-high heat) until it begins to turn lightly brown.
2. Combine the room-temperature butter, half of the shredded coconut, cinnamon, cardamom, and vanilla extract in a separate dish. Cool the mix in the fridge for about 5-10 minutes.
3. Form small balls and cover them with the remaining shredded coconut.
4. Cool the balls in the fridge for about 10-15 minutes.

Nutritions: *Carbohydrates – 0.4 g Fat – 10 g Protein – 0.4 g Calories – 90*

PREPARATION: 10 MIN **COOKING: 1H 35 MIN** **SERVES: 12**

EASY PEANUT BUTTER CUPS

INGREDIENTS

- 1/2 cup peanut butter
- 1/4 cup butter
- 3 oz. cacao butter, chopped
- 1/3 cup powdered swerve sweetener
- 1/2 tsp. vanilla extract
- 4 oz. sugar-free dark chocolate

DIRECTIONS

1. Line a muffin tin with parchment paper or cupcake liners.
2. Using low heat, melt the peanut butter, butter, and cacao butter in a saucepan. Stir them until completely combined.
3. Add the vanilla and sweetener until there are no more lumps.
4. Carefully place the mixture in the muffin cups.
5. Refrigerate it until firm.
6. Put chocolate in a bowl and set the bowl over boiling water. This is done to avoid direct contact with the heat. Stir the chocolate until completely melted.
7. Take the muffin out of the fridge and drizzle in the chocolate on top. Put it back again in the fridge to firm it up. This should take 15 minutes to finish.
8. Store and serve when needed.

Nutritions: *Calories: 200k Fat: 19g Carbohydrates: 6g Protein: 2.9g Fiber: 3.6g*

PREPARATION: 10 MIN **COOKING: 4 HOURS** **SERVES: 8**

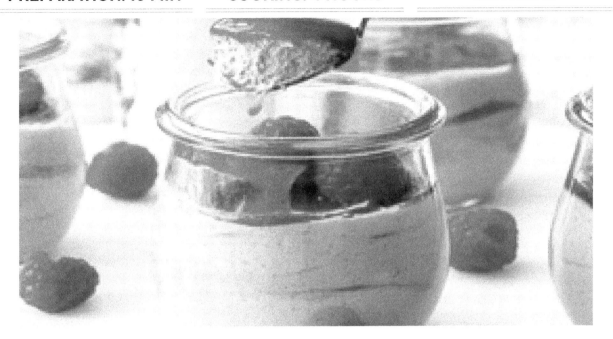

RASPBERRY MOUSSE

INGREDIENTS

- 3 oz. fresh raspberry
- 2 cups heavy whipping cream
- 2 oz. pecans, chopped
- ¼ tsp vanilla extract
- ½ lemon, the zest

DIRECTIONS

1. Pour the whipping cream into the dish and blend until it becomes soft.
2. Put the lemon zest and vanilla into the dish and mix thoroughly.
3. Put the raspberries and nuts into the cream mix and stir well.
4. Cover the dish with plastic wrap and put it in the fridge for 3 hours.
5. Top with raspberries and serve.

Nutritions: *Carbohydrates – 3 g Fat – 26 g Protein – 2 g Calories – 255*

PREPARATION: 5 MIN **COOKING: 5 MIN** **SERVES: 6**

CHOCOLATE SPREAD WITH HAZELNUTS

INGREDIENTS

- 2 Tbsp. cacao powder
- 5 oz. hazelnuts, roasted and without shells
- 1 oz. unsalted butter
- ¼ cup coconut oil

DIRECTIONS

1. Whisk all the spread ingredients with a blender for as long as you want. Remember, the longer you blend, the smoother your spread.

Nutritions: *Carbohydrates –2 g Fat – 28 g Protein – 4 g Calories – 271*

PREPARATION: 20 MIN **COOKING: 5 MIN** **SERVES: 2**

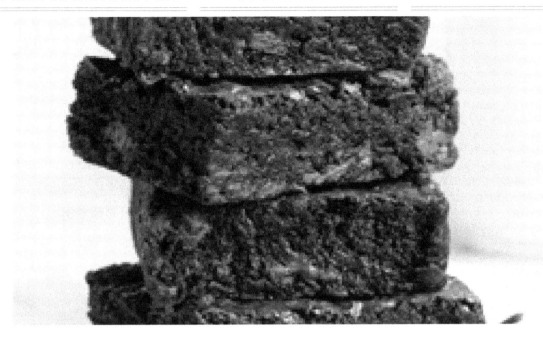

QUICK AND SIMPLE BROWNIE

INGREDIENTS

- 3 Tbsp. Keto chocolate chips
- 1 Tbsp. unsweetened cacao powder
- 2 Tbsp. salted butter
- 2¼ Tbsp. powdered sugar

DIRECTIONS

1. Combine 2 tbsp. of chocolate chips and butter, melt them in a microwave for 10-15 minutes. Add the remaining chocolate chips, stir and make a sauce.
2. Add the cacao powder and powdered sugar to the sauce and whisk well until you have a dough.
3. Place the dough on a baking sheet, form the brownie.
4. Put your brownie into the oven (preheated to 350°F).
5. Bake for 5 minutes.

Nutritions: *Carbohydrates – 9 g Fat – 30 g Protein – 13 g Calories – 100*

PREPARATION: 20 MIN **COOKING: 20 MIN** **SERVES: 18**

CUTE PEANUT BALLS

INGREDIENTS

- 1 cup salted peanuts, chopped
- 1 cup peanut butter
- 1 cup powdered sweetener
- 8 oz keto chocolate chips

DIRECTIONS

1. Combine the chopped peanuts, peanut butter, and sweetener in a separate dish. Stir well and make a dough. Divide it into 18 pieces and form small balls. Put them in the fridge for 10-15 minutes.
2. Use a microwave to melt your chocolate chips.
3. Plunge each ball into the melted chocolate.
4. Return your balls to the fridge. Cool for about 20 minutes.

Nutritions: *Carbohydrates – 7 g Fat – 17 g Protein – 7 g Calories – 194*

PREPARATION: 5 MIN **COOKING: 2 MIN** **SERVES: 4**

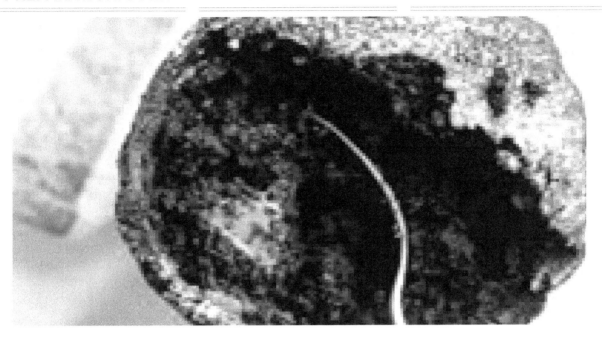

CHOCOLATE MUG MUFFINS

INGREDIENTS

- 4 tbsps. almond flour
- 1 tsp. baking powder
- 4 tbsp. granulated Erythritol
- 2 tbsp. cocoa powder
- ½ tsp. vanilla extract
- 2 pinches salt
- 2 eggs beaten
- 3 tbsp. butter, melted
- 1 tsp. coconut oil, for greasing the mug
- ½ oz. sugar-free dark chocolate, chopped

DIRECTIONS

1. Mix the dry ingredients together in a separate bowl. Add the melted butter, beaten eggs, and chocolate to the bowl. Stir thoroughly.
2. Divide your dough into 4 pieces. Put these pieces in the greased mugs and put them in the microwave. Cook for 1-1.5 minutes (700 watts).
3. Let them cool for 1 minute and serve.

Nutritions: *Carbohydrates – 2 g Fat – 19 g Protein – 5 g Calories – 208*

13. CONDIMENTS, SAUCES, & SPREADS RECIPES

Sometimes people associate the word "diet" with foods that taste bad, but just because you're following a specific eating plan doesn't mean your food shouldn't taste good. If you're used to adding sauces and dressings to all of your foods, it's easy to find keto versions of these seasonings to complement your dishes. Since many common seasonings contain added sugar or carbohydrates that are not part of the Keto diet, you will need to read the nutrition labels before buying anything! But don't be afraid – there are plenty of Keto condiments you can keep at home to spice up your meals.

When buying ingredients, it is also important to check the ingredient labels. We recommend that you buy minimally processed ingredients and use whole foods. Another option is to make your own toppings at home. Just mixing herbs and spices can produce flavorful, keto-safe seasonings, and you won't have to worry about adding sugars or other sweeteners.

If you are a fan of taco sauce or prefer an herb mix, there is a keto sauce for you. Here are a few you should always have in your pantry:

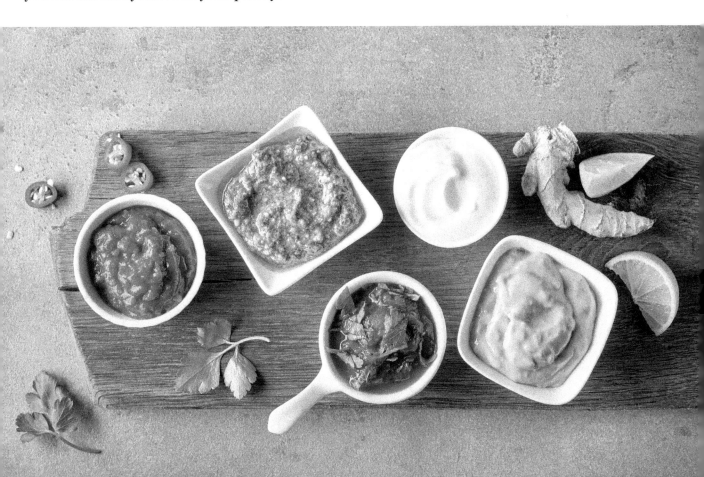

PREPARATION: 5 MIN **COOKING: 2 MIN** **SERVES: 4**

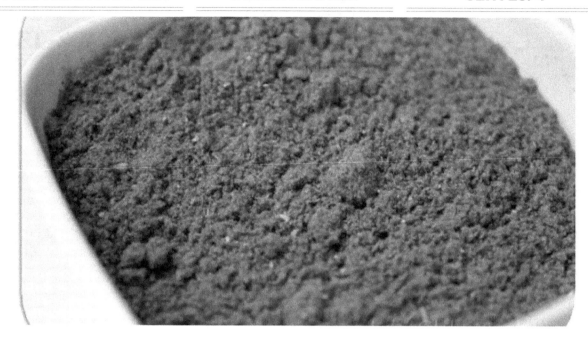

CURRY POWDER

INGREDIENTS

- ¼ cup coriander seeds
- 2 tablespoons mustard seeds
- 2 tablespoons cumin seeds
- 2 tablespoons anise seeds
- 1 tablespoon whole allspice berries
- 1 tablespoon fenugreek seeds
- 5 tablespoons ground turmeric

DIRECTIONS

1. In a large nonstick frying pan, place all the spices except turmeric over medium heat and cook for about 9–10 minutes or until toasted completely, stirring continuously.
2. Remove the frying pan from heat and set aside to cool.
3. In a spice grinder, add the toasted spices and turmeric, and grind until a fine powder forms.
4. Transfer to an airtight jar to preserve.

Nutritions: *Calories 18 Net Carbs 1.8 g Total Fat 0.8 g Saturated Fat 0.1 g Cholesterol 0 mg Sodium 3 mg Total Carbs 2.7 g Fiber 0.9 g Sugar 0.1 g Protein 0.8 g*

PREPARATION: 5 MIN **COOKING: 5 MIN** **SERVES: 10**

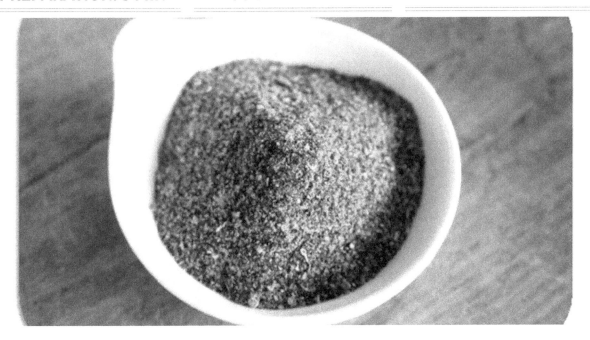

POULTRY SEASONING

INGREDIENTS

- 2 teaspoons dried sage, crushed finely
- 1 teaspoon dried marjoram, crushed finely
- ¾ teaspoon dried rosemary, crushed finely
- 1½ teaspoons dried thyme, crushed finely
- ½ teaspoon ground nutmeg
- ½ teaspoon ground black pepper

DIRECTIONS

1. Add all the ingredients to a bowl and stir to combine.
2. Transfer into an airtight jar to preserve.

Nutritions: *Calories 2 Net Carbs 0.2 g Total Fat 0.1g Saturated Fat 0.1 g Cholesterol 0 mg Sodium 0 mg Total Carbs 0.4 g Fiber 0.2 g Sugar 0 g Protein 0.1 g*

PREPARATION: 15 MIN   **COOKING: 20 MIN**   **SERVES: 20**

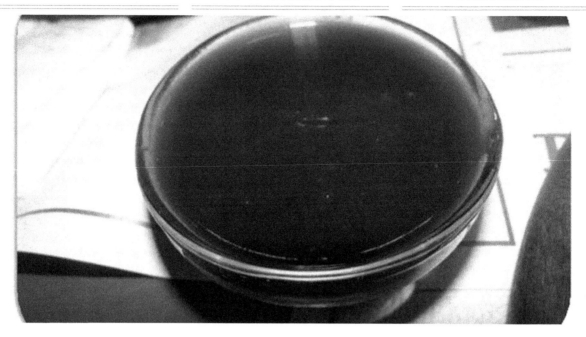

BBQ SAUCE

INGREDIENTS

- 2½ (6-ounces) cans sugar-free tomato paste
- ½ cup organic apple cider vinegar
- 1/3 cup powdered erythritol
- 2 tablespoons Worcestershire sauce
- 1 tablespoon liquid smoke
- 2 teaspoons smoked paprika
- 1 teaspoon garlic powder
- ½ teaspoon onion powder
- Salt, as required
- ¼ teaspoon red chili powder
- ¼ teaspoon cayenne pepper
- 1½ cups water

DIRECTIONS

1. Add all the ingredients (except the water) to a pan and beat until well combined.
2. Add 1 cup of water and beat until combined.
3. Add the remaining water and beat until well combined.
4. Place the pan over medium-high heat and bring to a gentle boil.
5. Adjust the heat to medium-low and simmer, uncovered for about 20 minutes, stirring frequently.
6. Remove the pan of sauce from the heat and set aside to cool slightly before serving.
7. You can preserve this sauce in the refrigerator by placing it into an airtight container

Nutritions: *Calories 22 Net Carbs 3.7 g Total Fat 0.1 g Saturated Fat 0 g Cholesterol 0 mg Sodium 46 mg Total Carbs 4.7 g Fiber 1 g Sugar 3 g Protein 1 g*

PREPARATION: 10 MIN **COOKING: 30 MIN** **SERVES: 12**

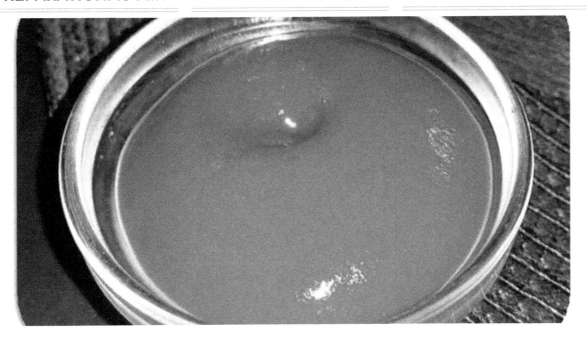

KETCHUP

INGREDIENTS

- 6 ounces sugar-free tomato paste
- 1 cup of water
- ¼ cup powdered erythritol
- 3 tablespoons balsamic vinegar
- ½ teaspoon garlic powder
- ½ teaspoon onion powder
- ¼ teaspoon paprika
- 1/8 teaspoon ground cloves
- 1/8 teaspoon mustard powder
- Salt, as required

DIRECTIONS

1. Add all ingredients in a small pan and beat until smooth.
2. Now, place the pan over medium heat and bring to a gentle simmer, stirring continuously.
3. Adjust the heat to low and simmer, covered for about 30 minutes or until desired thickness, stirring occasionally.
4. Remove the pan from heat, and with an immersion blender, blend until smooth.
5. Now, set aside to cool completely before serving.
6. You can preserve this ketchup in the refrigerator by placing it in an airtight container.

Nutritions: *Calories 13 Net Carbs 2.3 g Total Fat 0.1 g Saturated Fat 0 g Cholesterol 0 mg Sodium 26 mg Total Carbs 2.9 g Fiber 0.6 g Sugar 1.8 g Protein 0.7 g*

PREPARATION: 10 MIN **COOKING: 15 MIN** **SERVES: 6**

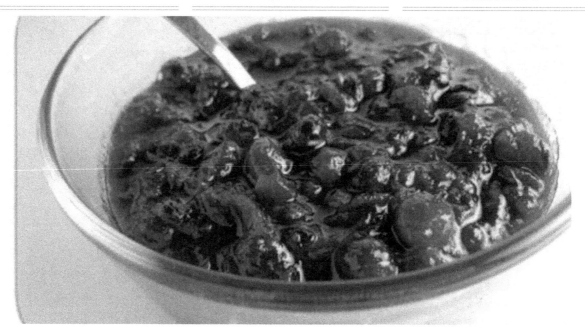

CRANBERRY SAUCE

INGREDIENTS

- 12 ounces fresh cranberries
- 1 cup powdered erythritol
- ¾ cup of water
- 1 teaspoon fresh lemon zest, grated
- ½ teaspoon organic vanilla extract

DIRECTIONS

1. Place the cranberries, water, erythritol, and lemon zest in a medium pan and mix well.
2. Place the pan over medium heat and bring to a boil.
3. Adjust the heat to low and simmer for about 12–15 minutes, stirring frequently.
4. Remove the pan from heat and mix in the vanilla extract.
5. Set aside at room temperature to cool completely.
6. Transfer the sauce into a bowl and refrigerate to chill before serving.

Nutritions: *Calories 32 Net Carbs 3.2 g Total Fat 0 g Saturated Fat 0 g Cholesterol 0 mg Sodium 1 mg Total Carbs 5.3 g Fiber 2.1 g Sugar 2.1 g Protein 0 g*

PREPARATION: 10 MIN **COOKING: 30 MIN** **SERVES: 12**

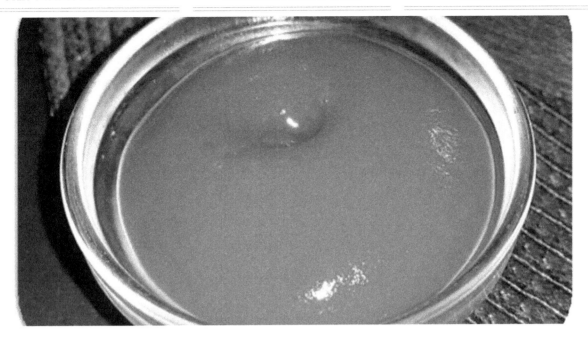

KETCHUP

INGREDIENTS

- 6 ounces sugar-free tomato paste
- 1 cup of water
- ¼ cup powdered erythritol
- 3 tablespoons balsamic vinegar
- ½ teaspoon garlic powder
- ½ teaspoon onion powder
- ¼ teaspoon paprika
- 1/8 teaspoon ground cloves
- 1/8 teaspoon mustard powder
- Salt, as required

DIRECTIONS

1. Add all ingredients in a small pan and beat until smooth.
2. Now, place the pan over medium heat and bring to a gentle simmer, stirring continuously.
3. Adjust the heat to low and simmer, covered for about 30 minutes or until desired thickness, stirring occasionally.
4. Remove the pan from heat, and with an immersion blender, blend until smooth.
5. Now, set aside to cool completely before serving.
6. You can preserve this ketchup in the refrigerator by placing it in an airtight container.

Nutritions: *Calories 13 Net Carbs 2.3 g Total Fat 0.1 g Saturated Fat 0 g Cholesterol 0 mg Sodium 26 mg Total Carbs 2.9 g Fiber 0.6 g Sugar 1.8 g Protein 0.7 g*

PREPARATION: 10 MIN **COOKING: 0 MIN** **SERVES: 3**

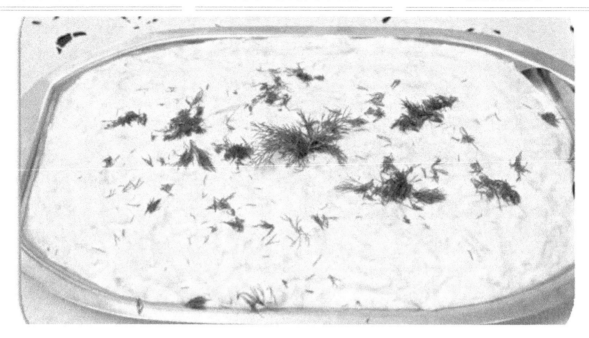

YOGURT TZATZIKI

INGREDIENTS

- 1 large English cucumber, peeled and grated
- Salt, as required
- 2 cups plain Greek yogurt
- 1 tablespoon fresh lemon juice
- 4 garlic cloves, minced
- 1 tablespoon fresh mint leaves, chopped
- 2 tablespoons fresh dill, chopped
- Pinch of cayenne pepper
- Ground black pepper, as required

DIRECTIONS

1. Arrange a colander in the sink.
2. Place the cucumber into the colander and sprinkle with salt.
3. Let it drain for about 10–15 minutes.
4. With your hands, squeeze the cucumber well.
5. Place the cucumber and remaining ingredients in a large bowl and stir to combine.
6. Cover the bowl and place in the refrigerator to chill for at least 4–8 hours before serving.

Nutritions: *Calories 36 Net Carbs 4.2 g Total Fat 0.6 g Saturated Fat 0.4 g Cholesterol 2 mg Sodium 42 mg Total Carbs 4.5 g Fiber 0.3 g Sugar 3.3 g Protein 2.7 g*

14. 30-DAY MEAL PLAN

Day	Breakfast	Lunch	Snack	Dinner	Dessert
1	Almond Coconut Egg Wraps	Turkey & Cream Cheese Sauce	Parmesan Cheese Strips	Baked Zucchini Noodles with Feta	Sugar-free Lemon Bars
2	Bacon & Avocado Omelet	Baked Salmon & Pesto	Peanut Butter Power Granola	Brussels Sprouts with Bacon	Creamy Hot Chocolate
3	Bacon & Cheese Frittata	Keto Chicken with Butter & Lemon	Homemade Graham Crackers	Bunless Burger- Keto Style	Delicious Coffee Ice cream
4	Bacon & Egg Breakfast Muffins	Garlic Chicken	Keto no Bake Cookies	Coffee BBQ Pork Belly	Fatty Bombs with Cinnamon and Cardamom
5	Bacon Hash	Salmon Skewers & Wrapped with Prosciutto	Swiss Cheese Crunchy Nachos	Garlic & Thyme Lamb Chops	Raspberry Mousse
6	Bagel with Cheese	Buffalo Drumsticks & Chili Aioli	Homemade Thin Mints	Jamaican Jerk Pork Roast	Quick & Simple Brownie
7	Baked Apples	Slow Cooked Roasted Pork & Creamy Gravy	Mozzarella Cheese Pockets	Keto Meatballs	Cute Peanut Balls
8	Baked Eggs in the Avocado	Bacon-Wrapped Meatloaf	No bake coconut Cookies	Mixed Vegetable patties- Instant pot	Chocolate Mug Muffins
9	Banana Pancakes	Lamb Chops & Herb Butter	Cheesy Cauliflower Breadsticks	Roasted Leg of Lamb	Chocolate Spreads with Hazelnuts

10	Breakfast Skillet	Crispy Cuban Pork Roast	Easy Peanut Butter Cups	Salmon Pasta	Keto Peanut Butter Cup Style Fudge
11	Brunch BLT Wrap	Keto Barbecued Ribs	Fried Green Beans Rosemary	Skillet Fried Cod	Keto and dairy-free Vanilla Custard
12	Cheesy Bacon & Egg Cups	Turkey Burgers & Tomato Butter	Crispy Broccoli Popcorn	Slow-Cooked Kalua Pork & Cabbage	Keto Triple Chocolate Mug Cake
13	Coconut Keto Porridge	Keto Hamburger	Cheesy Cauliflower Croquettes	Steak Pinwheels	Keto Cheesecake Stuffed Brownies
14	Cream Cheese Eggs	Chicken wings & Blue Cheese Dressing	Spinach in Cheese Envelopes	Tangy Shrimp	Keto Raspberry Ice cream
15	Creamy Basil Baked Sausage	Salmon Burgers with Lemon Butter & Mash	Cheesy Mushroom Slices	Chicken Salad with Champagne Vinegar	Chocolate Macadamia Nut Fat Bombs
16	Banana Waffles	Egg Salad Recipe	Asparagus Fries	Mexican Beef Salad	Keto Peanut Butter Chocolate Bars
17	Keto Cinnamon Coffee	Taco Stuffed Avocados	Kale Chips	Cherry Tomatoes Tilapia Salad	Salted Toffee Nut Cups
18	Keto Waffles & Blueberries	Buffalo Shrimp Lettuce Wraps	Guacamole	Crunchy Chicken Milanese	Crisp Meringue Cookies
19	Baked Avocado Eggs	Broccoli Bacon Salad	Zucchini Noodles	Parmesan Baked Chicken	Instant Pot Matcha Cookies
20	Mushroom Omelet	Keto Egg Salad	Cauliflower Souffle	Cheesy Bacon and Broccoli Chicken	Matcha Skillet Souffle

21	Chocolate Sea Salt Smoothie	Loaded Cauliflower Salad	No-Churn Ice Cream	Buttery Garlic Chicken	Flourless Keto Brownies
22	Zucchini Lasagna	Caprese Zoodles	Cheesecake Cupcakes	Creamy Slow Cooker Chicken	Tropical Chocolate Mousse Bites
23	Vegan Keto Scramble	Zucchini Sushi	Chocolate Peanut Butter Cups	Braised Chicken Thighs with Kalamata Olives	Coconut Raspberry Slice
24	Bavarian Cream with Vanilla and Hazelnuts	Asian Chicken Lettuce Wraps	Low-carb Almond Coconut Sandies	Baked Garlic and Paprika Chicken Legs	White Chocolate Bark
25	Vanilla Mousse	California Burger Bowls	Crème Brulee	Chicken Curry with Masala	Keto Hot Chocolate
26	Blueberry Mousse	Parmesan Brussels Sprouts Salad	Chocolate Fat Bomb	Chicken Quesadilla	Carrot Cake Chia Pudding
27	Strawberry Bavarian	Chicken Taco Avocados	Cocoa Mug Cake	Slow Cooker BBQ Ribs	Carrot Cake Energy Balls
28	Almond mousse	Keto Quesadillas	Dark Chocolate Espresso Paleo & Keto mug Cake	Barbacoa Beef Roast	Caramel Pecan Muffins
29	Nougat	No-bread Italian Subs	Keto Matcha Mint Bars	Beef & Broccoli Roast	Cinnamon Roll Cookies
30	Chocolate Crepes	Basil Avocado frail Salad Wraps & Sweet Potato Chips	Keto No-churn blueberry Maple Ice cream	Cauliflower and Pumpkin Casserole	Zucchini Cookies

15. PROHIBITED PRODUCTS LIST

Because the diet is a Keto diet, that means you need to avoid high-carb food. Some of the food you avoid is even healthy, but it just contains too many carbs. Here is a list of typical food you should limit or avoid altogether.

Bread and Grains

No matter what form bread takes, they still pack a lot of carbs. The same applies to whole-grain as well because they are made from refined flour. So, if you want to eat bread, it is best to make keto variants at home instead.

Grains such as rice, wheat, and oats pack a lot of carbs as well. So, limit or avoid that as well.

Fruits

Fruits are healthy for you. The problem is that some of those foods pack quite a lot of carbs such as banana, raisins, dates, mango, and pear. As a general rule, avoid sweet and dried fruits.

Vegetables

Vegetables are just as healthy for your body. For one, they make you feel full for longer, so they help suppress your appetite. But that also means you need to avoid or limit vegetables that are high in starch because they have more carbs than fiber. That includes corn, potato, sweet potato, and beets.

Pasta

As with any other convenient food, pasta is rich in carbs. So, spaghetti or any different types of pasta are not recommended when you are on your keto diet.

Cereal

Cereal is also a considerable offender because sugary breakfast cereals pack a lot of carbs. That also applies to "healthy cereals." Just because they use other words to describe their product does not mean that you should believe them. That also applies to oatmeal, whole-grain cereals, etc.

Beer

In reality, you can drink most alcoholic beverages in moderation without fear. Beer is an exception to this rule because it packs a lot of carbs. Carbs in beers or other liquids are considered liquid carbs, and they are even more dangerous than substantial carbs.

Sweetened Yogurt

Yogurt is very healthy because it is tasty and does not have that many carbs. The problem comes when you consume yogurt variants rich in carbs such as fruit-flavored, low-fat, sweetened, or nonfat yogurt. A single serving of sweetened yogurt contains as many carbs as a single serving of dessert.

Juice

Fruit juices are perhaps the worst beverage you can put into your system when you are on a keto diet. Another problem is that the brain does not process liquid carbs the same way as stable carbs. Substantial carbs can help suppress appetite, but liquid carbs will only put your need into overdrive.

Low-Fat and Fat-Free Salad Dressings

If you have to buy salads, keep in mind that commercial sauces pack more carbs than you think, especially the fat-free and low-fat variants.

Beans and Legumes

These are also very nutritious as they are rich in fiber. However, they are also rich in carbs. You may enjoy a small amount of them when you are on your Keto diet, but don't exceed your carb limit.

Sugar

We mean sugar in any form, including honey. Foods that contain lots of sugar, such as cookies, candies, and cake, are forbidden on a Keto diet or any other form of diet that is designed to lose weight. When you are on a Keto diet, you need to keep in mind that your diet consists of food that is rich in fiber and nutritious. So, sugar is out of the question.

Chips and Crackers

These two are some of the most popular snacks. Some people did not realize that one packet of chips contains several servings and should not be all eaten in one go. The carbs can add up very quickly if you do not watch what you eat.

Milk

Milk also contains a lot of carbs on its own. Therefore, avoid it if you can, even though milk is a good source of many nutrients such as calcium, potassium, and other B vitamins.

Gluten-Free Baked Goods

Gluten-free diets are trendy nowadays, but what many people don't seem to realize is that they pack quite a lot of carbs. That includes gluten-free bread, muffins, and other baked products. In reality, they contain even more carbs than their glutenous variant.

CONCLUSION

Now that you are familiar with the Keto diet on many levels, you should feel confident in your ability to start your own Keto journey. This diet plan isn't going to hinder you or limit you, so do your best to keep this in mind as you begin changing your lifestyle and adjusting your eating habits. Packed with good fats and plenty of protein, your body is going to go through a transformation as it works to see these things as energy. Before you know it, your body will have an automatically accessible reserve that you can utilize at any time. Whether you need a boost of energy first thing in the morning or a second wind to keep you going throughout the day, this will already be inside of you.

As you take care of yourself through the next few years, you can feel great knowing that the Keto diet aligns with the anti-aging lifestyle that you seek. Not only does it keep you looking great and feeling younger, but it also acts as a preventative barrier from various ailments and conditions. The body tends to weaken as you age, but Keto helps to keep a shield up in front of it by giving you plenty of opportunities to burn energy and create muscle mass. Instead of taking the things that you need to feel great, Keto only takes what you have in abundance. This is how you will always end up feeling your best each day.

Arguably one of the best diets around, Keto keeps you feeling so great because you have many meal options! There is no shortage of delicious and filling meals that you can eat while you are on any of the Keto diet plans. You can even take this diet with you as you eat out at restaurants and friends' houses. As long as you can remember the simple guidelines, you should have no problems staying on track with Keto. Cravings become almost non-existent as your body works to change the way it digests. Instead of relying on glucose in your bloodstream, your body switches focus. It begins using fat as soon as you reach the state of ketosis that you are aiming for. The best part is you do not have to do anything other than eating within your fat/protein/carb percentages. Your body will do the rest on its own.

Because this is a way that your body can properly function for long periods, Keto is proven to be more than a simple fad diet. Originating with a medical background for helping epilepsy patients, the Keto diet has been tried and tested for decades. Many successful studies align with the knowledge that Keto works. Whether you are trying to be on a diet for a month or a year, both are just as healthy for you. Keto is an adjustment, but it is one that will continue benefiting you for as long as you are able to keep it up. Good luck on your journey ahead!

CPSIA information can be obtained
at www.ICGtesting.com
Printed in the USA
LVHW101923030321
680491LV00007B/211